Domestic Violence and Mental Health

T0203280

Edited by Louise M. Howard, Gene Feder
and Roxane Agnew-Davies

RCPsych Publications

© The Royal College of Psychiatrists 2013

RCPsych Publications is an imprint of the Royal College of Psychiatrists,
17 Belgrave Square, London SW1X 8PG
http://www.rcpsych.ac.uk

British Library Cataloguing-in-Publication Data.
A catalogue record for this book is available from the British Library.
ISBN 978 1 908020 56 7

Distributed in North America by Publishers Storage and Shipping Company.

Printed by Bell & Bain Limited, Glasgow, UK.

Contents

Tables, boxes and figures

Contributors

Roxane Agnew-Davies C Psychol, AFBPsS   Director, Domestic Violence Training Ltd, Mental Health Advisor, AVA (Against Violence & Abuse), and Honorary Research Fellow, Department of Social and Community Medicine, University of Bristol

Gene Feder   Professor of Primary Health Care, School of Social and Community Medicine, University of Bristol

Louise M. Howard   Head of Section for Women's Mental Health, Institute of Psychiatry, King's College London

Emma Howarth   Research Associate, School of Social and Community Medicine, University of Bristol

Fiona Mason MB BS FRCPsych DFP   Chief Medical Officer, St Andrew's Healthcare, and Associate Registrar Leadership and Management, Royal College of Psychiatrists

Siân Oram   Researcher, Institute of Psychiatry, King's College London

Kylee Trevillion   Researcher, Institute of Psychiatry, King's College London

CHAPTER 1

Prevalence and physical health impact of domestic violence

Emma Howarth and Gene Feder

Domestic violence and abuse is threatening behaviour, violence or abuse between adults who are relatives, partners or ex-partners. It includes abuse from adult children and from parents of adult children. Domestic violence is a breach of human rights as well as a major public health and clinical problem. In this chapter we focus largely on violence between partners or ex-partners when discussing prevalence, and exclusively on partner violence when reviewing evidence on the health impact of domestic violence and abuse, as this is the focus of most research to date.

Definition of intimate partner violence

Intimate partner violence is a form of domestic violence occurring between intimate partners or ex-partners. Whereas violence between partners occurs in all types of relationships and cuts across all sections of society, intimate partner violence is recognised as a gendered issue where women are overwhelmingly more likely to be injured as a result of violence, require medical attention or hospital admission, and fear for their lives, and men are more likely to perpetrate violence. Internationally, there are no consistent demographic associations with intimate partner violence, such as ethnicity, age and number of children, other than relative poverty. Although it is prevalent across the socioeconomic spectrum, intimate partner violence is more common in families and communities which are relatively deprived (Pickett & Wilkinson, 2009). In the UK, the USA and Canada, younger women (aged between 16 and 34) experience the highest rates of intimate partner violence (Smith *et al*, 2011; Catalano, 2012; Sinha, 2012) and there is some evidence that women with disabilities are at increased risk (Mirlees-Black, 1999).

In earlier decades, terms such as wife abuse, conjugal violence and spousal abuse were commonplace, but they have been superseded by more general terms, such as domestic violence, in recognition that violence and abuse does not just occur between married couples. In the UK, domestic violence has a precise definition denoting violence between adults who are relatives, partners or ex-partners (Home Office, 2012). Intimate partner violence specifically refers to abuse from partners or ex-partners, distinguishing it from other forms of violence that may occur in a family or domestic setting. The World Health Organization (WHO) defines intimate partner violence broadly, as any behaviour within an intimate relationship that causes physical, psychological or sexual harm to those in the relationship; it includes: physical aggression, psychological abuse, forced intercourse and other forms of sexual coercion, as well as various controlling behaviours (Krug *et al*, 2002*a*). This definition reflects the increasingly recognised multidimensional nature of intimate partner violence where physical abuse is just one part of the pattern of abusive behaviour that individuals may experience. Examples of the types of behaviour that fall within the scope of intimate partner violence are outlined below.

Physical abuse

Physical violence is included in most definitions of intimate partner violence (Nicolaidis & Paranjape, 2009), although as discussed below different disciplines may place more or less emphasis on minor forms of violence. Conceptualisations of physical violence may include:
- hitting, slapping, pushing, kicking
- the use of weapons or objects as weapons
- burning, scalding
- choking
- hair-pulling
- interference with medical treatment
- undue restraint or inappropriate sanctions.

Sexual abuse

Sexual abuse includes (Abraham, 1999; Bacchus *et al*, 2006):
- rape, attempted rape and sexual assault
- coerced sexual contact
- being forced to watch or re-enact pornographic material
- denial of the right to use contraception.

Psychological abuse

Psychological abuse includes (Follingstad *et al*, 1990):
- reoccurring criticism
- verbal aggression
- jealous behaviour and accusations of infidelity
- threats of violence
- threats to end the relationship
- hostile withdrawal of affection
- destroying property.

Research shows that psychological abuse can have severe consequences, even after controlling for the effects of physical abuse (Marshall, 1996;

Arias & Pape, 1999), and many victims of intimate partner violence rate the impact of emotional abuse on their lives as more profound than that of the physical abuse (Follingstad *et al*, 1990; Murphy & Hoover, 1999; O'Leary, 1999; Coker *et al*, 2000).

Coercive control

Some researchers conceptualise coercive control rather than physical violence as the defining feature of intimate partner abuse (Johnson, 1995, 2006; Dutton & Goodman, 2005). In this vein, Hegarty (2006) argues that it may be more useful from a health perspective to conceive of intimate partner violence as a 'chronic syndrome' that is characterised not by the episodes of physical violence that punctuate it, but by the range of behaviours including emotional and psychological abuse that perpetrators invoke to exert and maintain control over their partners. The level of control exerted by one party over another is argued by some to distinguish relationships that are simply conflicted and occasionally violent from those which are abusive (Johnson, 1995, 2006; Gordon, 2000; Carbone-Lopez *et al*, 2006) and which characterise the experiences of a large proportion of victims who make contact with specialist domestic violence services (Graham-Kevan & Archer, 2003*a,b*; Carbone-Lopez *et al*, 2006; Johnson, 2006). On the other hand, others consider all acts of violence as intimate partner violence (Straus, 1990). These differences in conceptualisation may be a function of discipline and the theoretical perspective held by researchers.

Controlling behaviour may manifest as (McCloskey, 2001; Beeble *et al*, 2007):

(a) isolation from friends, family and other support networks;
(b) limited access to money;
(c) surveillance of everyday tasks such as grocery shopping;
(d) intercepting mail, phone calls and text messages;
(e) threats to harm or kill children.

Harassment and stalking may also form part of a general pattern of coercion and control, although these behaviours are sometimes regarded as distinct from one another (e.g. Tjaden & Thoennes, 1998; Britton, 2012). Common stalking behaviours include unwanted communication (phone calls, text messages or emails), being followed on the street, contacted at home or at work, unwelcome visits or gifts, threats, damage to property, violence, and gaining information about the victim under false pretences, for example posing as a family member (Abrams & Robinson, 1998; Kamphuis & Emmelkamp, 2001).

Definitional issues

The myriad definitions of intimate partner violence that conceptualise it in slightly different ways complicate comparisons between epidemiological studies measuring prevalence and impact. Therefore, before turning to a discussion of prevalence we consider some of the issues that may determine the way that intimate partner violence is defined, and which may in part account for differences in prevalence rates and estimates of impact (Alhabib *et al*, 2010).

The definition of intimate partner violence that we use throughout this book captures its multidimensional nature, encompassing non-physical forms of abuse in recognition of their impact on individuals' health and well-being. Others are narrower and consider only physical acts of violence (e.g. Straus, 1986; Rodgers, 1994) or emotional abuse in the context of physical violence (e.g. Saltzman *et al*, 2002). The decision to include one, some or all of the components of abuse outlined earlier can differ from researcher to researcher and discipline to discipline (Gordon, 2000).

Different disciplines have different goals, objectives and methods of research (Desai & Saltzman, 2001; Nicolaidis & Paranjape, 2009), which undoubtedly affects the way that abuse is defined. Family conflict researchers, who consider violence to be a response to conflict, define intimate partner violence as any abusive act perpetrated by men or women, with less consideration of antecedents to violence, intent and consequences (e.g. Straus, 1997; Archer, 2000), or the use of non-violent tactics. In contrast, feminist researchers, placing emphasis on the power dynamics of the relationship as well as intent and consequences, use broader definitions (e.g. Stark & Buzawa, 2009). Based on these two disparate perspectives, an isolated slap that is enacted in the 'heat of the moment' and does not form part of a wider pattern of behavior may be considered abusive by family conflict researchers, but not those subscribing to a feminist perspective (Hegarty, 2006; Nicolaidis & Paranjape, 2009).

Definitions further vary in terms of their reference to the impact of the abuse. The WHO definition, along with several others, makes reference to the impact of behaviour, with only that which causes harm defined as violence (e.g. Weis, 1989); others do not make any particular reference, instead focusing simply on the frequency and severity of behaviours, although it is worth noting that frequent but more minor acts may be just as damaging to an individual's physical and emotional health as a more severe but one-off violent act (Gordon, 2000; Hegarty, 2006). Consideration of harm caused may be a good way of encompassing all behaviours, minor and major, that comprise abuse, and also of giving some weight to the context in which the behaviour occurs, given that the emotional impact of behaviours may depend on factors such as past abuse (Mahoney *et al*, 2001). Further, not all violent acts are equal (Mahoney *et al*, 2001) and appraisal of harm may also be a way by which the same acts perpetrated by men and women can be classified differently, given that the same act perpetrated by a man may have a greater impact than if perpetrated by a woman (Dobash *et al*, 1992). However, it may be more difficult to make this distinction for non-physical acts. Several authors suggest that definitions of violence should include the intent with which behaviour is carried out (Burke *et al*, 1989; Weis, 1989; Hegarty, 2006), which may help to determine what constitutes abuse, although Hegarty (2006) points out that this is a facet rarely reflected in definitions and measurement of abuse.

In summary, how intimate partner violence is defined determines how it is measured and in turn, determines conclusions about its nature and magnitude (Waltermaurer, 2005; Nicolaidis & Paranjape, 2009; Alhabib *et al*, 2010). Studies which adopt broader definitions of abuse yield higher rates than those which use narrower definitions; those undertaken from a family conflict perspective which focus on the frequency of discrete behaviours suggest that rates of partner violence perpetration are comparable between men and women; whereas other studies considering the severity, intentions and impact of violence reveal significant gender asymmetry. These are issues of which one needs to be aware when appraising estimates of prevalence, although understanding whether variation in rates reflects true difference or can in part be attributed to a difference in definition is made difficult by the fact that few studies even describe the criteria used to define the abused sample (Geffner *et al*, 1988; Alhabib *et al*, 2010).

Prevalence

Prevalence studies estimate the proportion of a population that has suffered intimate partner violence during adult life or during a specified time period. They are important in understanding the scale of the problem (Heise *et al*, 1999; Walby & Myhill 2001; Krug *et al*, 2002*b*), although, as outlined earlier, variation between studies may reflect a combination of real and measurement differences. Further, the population sampled may also have a bearing on estimates derived from studies, with clinical populations tending to yield the highest rates (Feder *et al*, 2009; Alhabib *et al*, 2010).

Between 2000 and 2003, the WHO undertook a multicountry study with the aim of estimating the extent of physical and sexual intimate partner violence against women in 15 sites in ten countries (Bangladesh, Brazil, Ethiopia, Japan, Namibia, Peru, Samoa, Serbia and Montenegro, Thailand, and the United Republic of Tanzania). This study, with 24 000 participants aged 14 to 59 years and using standardised survey methods, is to date the most robust comparison between countries, although figures do not represent national prevalence rates because the samples were based in specific rural or urban settings (Garcia-Moreno *et al*, 2006).

The reported lifetime prevalence of physical or sexual violence, or both, for ever-partnered women varied from 15 to 71%; and the 12-month prevalence rates in the sample varied from 4 to 54%. The percentage of ever-partnered women in the population who had experienced severe physical violence ranged from 4% in a Japanese city to 49% in a province in Peru. The proportion of women reporting one or more acts of their partners' controlling behaviour (including keeping from family and friends, expecting a woman to seek permission before seeking medical treatment) ranged from 21 to 90%. With respect to this finding, the authors suggest that these wide-ranging rates may reflect cultural differences with regard to the normative level of control in intimate relationships. However, the finding that women across all sites who suffered physical or sexual partner violence were substantially more likely to experience severe controlling behaviours than non-abused women is in line with the view that coercive control is a defining feature of intimate partner violence, irrespective of culture (Garcia-Moreno *et al*, 2006). Moreover, this study revealed consistent health consequences of intimate partner violence (see pp. 10–13 of this chapter), supporting the WHO's reference to the impact of abusive behaviour in their definition of intimate partner violence.

The British Crime Survey

In the UK, the British Crime Survey (BCS) is the most reliable source of community prevalence estimates. It is a face-to-face victimisation survey of over 40000 individuals aged between 16 and 59 in which people resident in households in England and Wales are asked about their experience of a range of crimes in the 12 months prior to the interview. The BCS is the best source for assessing long-term trends since it uses a consistent methodology and is not based on changes in reporting and recording procedures that can have an impact on criminal justice data. It is undertaken on a rolling basis, allowing comparisons of crime trends year on year. Intimate partner abuse is assessed using a self-completion module which asks respondents about their experiences of domestic abuse, sexual assault and stalking.

The 2010–2011 BCS reports lifetime partner abuse prevalence at 27% for women and 14% for men; 7% and 5% respectively had experienced abuse in the previous 12 months. The definition of partner abuse includes non-physical abuse, threats, force, sexual assault or stalking. The BCS also measures non-partner domestic violence (termed 'family abuse'), reporting a lifetime prevalence of 10% and 7% for women and men respectively. The starkest gender difference in prevalence revealed by the BCS is for sexual assault: 17% and 2% lifetime prevalence for women and men respectively, although these figures include assaults by partners, ex-partners, family members, or any other person. Examination of violent incidents recorded in the BCS (Hall & Innes, 2010) gives some sense of how common domestic abuse is compared with other types of violent victimisation. Data indicate that the majority of violent incidents against women are carried out by partners, ex-partners, family members (30%) or acquaintances (33%) as compared with 24% by strangers or 19% in mugging incidents. In contrast, the majority of incidents against men is categorised as stranger victimisation (44%) or mugging (19%); 6% as domestic and 32% acquaintance. Thus, the majority of violent incidents against women are carried out by people women know whereas for men violent incidents are most likely perpetrated by strangers.

Although the BCS represents the UK's best estimate of prevalence, there are two major caveats about its scope and measurement. First, the sampling frame excludes individuals living in 'institutional' settings including women's refuges. Unsurprisingly, samples based on women who have gone to refuges and shelters have consistently shown much higher frequency of abuse than those from national surveys (Dobash & Dobash, 1979; Okun, 1986; Straus, 1990), and this omission may have a particular impact on estimates of 12-month prevalence rates. The BCS also omits hospital in-patients, people living in hostels and people with no fixed abode; all of these groups are likely to have a higher exposure to domestic violence. Second, the BCS measures the frequency with which individuals experience any abusive acts, without consideration of the wider context in which these behaviours take place, creating a misleading picture of relative gender symmetry (Dobash *et al*, 1992). Using data from the 2001 survey, Walby & Allen (2004) demonstrated that women as compared with men were more likely to sustain some form of physical or psychological injury as a result of the worst incident experienced since the age of 16 (75% *v*. 50% physical; 37% *v*. 10% psychological), and more likely to experience severe injury such as broken bones (8% *v*. 2%) and severe bruising (21% *v*. 5%). Moreover, 89% of those reporting four or more incidents of domestic abuse were women. Whereas women are more likely than men to be the victims of escalated life-threatening levels of abuse, it is noted that where men do experience this type of violence it appears similar in its form and impact to that experienced by women (Carbone-Lopez *et al*, 2006; Johnson, 2006). Gender asymmetry is confirmed in other epidemiological studies, such as the Canadian Social Survey (Brennan, 2011), which found that a larger proportion of women reported being beaten, choked, threatened with or assaulted with a weapon by their partner in the past 5 years than did men (34% *v*. 10%) and women were more likely to state that they were injured as a result of the violence (42% *v*. 18%). This survey also found that the rate of spousal violence among those who are gay or lesbian was more than twice the rate of reported violence experienced by those who are heterosexual.

In north America, repeated cross-sectional population studies using the same methodology suggest that there has been a reduction over time in physical and sexual violence against women from their partners or ex-partners. For example, the 2004 Canadian Social Survey found a reduction of the 5-year prevalence of intimate partner violence against women from 8 to 7%, with the difference driven by reduction in intimate partner violence from ex-partners (AuCoin, 2005); rates remained stable between 2004 and 2009 (Brennan, 2011). In the UK, the BCS has shown a reduction of any current (past year) domestic abuse against women from 9% in 2004/2005 to 7% in 2010/2011 (Britton, 2012). This decline has been interpreted as a shift away from criminal acts to other methods of coercive control of women by their male partners or ex-partners, which may have similar impact on their long-term health (Stark, 2009). However, it has also been suggested that this reduction is in part accounted for by the development and increased utilisation of public services (Walby, 2009).

Women who currently experience or have a history of abuse use healthcare services more frequently than those with no history of abuse

(Bonomi *et al*, 2009). Therefore it is not surprising that the prevalence of intimate partner violence is higher in clinical than in community populations. A systematic review of 16 UK intimate partner violence prevalence studies (5 community and 11 clinical populations) found that both 1-year and lifetime prevalence were consistently lower in community populations: 75% lower for 1-year prevalence and 25% lower for lifetime prevalence (Feder *et al*, 2009). In a global systematic review of 134 prevalence studies, half representing community and half clinical populations, Alhabib *et al* (2010) found the highest prevalence of intimate partner violence in psychiatric and gynaecology clinics and in accident and emergency departments.

Causation

There is a profusion of competing theories attempting to explain intimate partner violence, each embedded in explanatory frameworks (Wolfe & Jaffe, 1999; Mitchell & Vanya, 2009). Within a psychological framework, early victim-blaming frustration–aggression theories were superseded by social learning and cognitive–behavioural theories. Within a biological framework, there are weak genetic influences on personality and cognitive traits associated with violence and there are strong neurohumoral and immunological mediators of violence on health. Within a sociological framework, economic relationships and cultural norms are seen to be playing a crucial role in reinforcing (or challenging) intimate partner violence. Within a feminist framework, intimate partner violence against women is construed as a form of social control that results from society's patriarchal structure leading to inequality in power relationships between men and women, a 'liberty crime' (Stark, 2009). The feminist framework has informed the human rights perspective on domestic violence.

The notion that perpetration of intimate partner violence was simply a function of psychopathology evaporated when it was found that most perpetrators do not have a personality disorder or a serious mental illness, although many abusive males have deficits in one or more of coping mechanisms, anger control and communication skills. The fact that male perpetrators and female victims are more likely to report histories of exposure to violence in childhood supports this theory. Although there appears to be an important transmission effect, most individuals exposed to violence do not commit violence as adults, and not all who do abuse have had a violent upbringing. Furthermore, the link between poor parenting, including neglect, and subsequent intimate partner violence in adulthood suggests that the effect is not simply one of modelling abusive behaviour. Exposure to rejecting or neglectful parenting is associated with adverse effects on intrapersonal (e.g. poor self-worth) and interpersonal development, which are associated with intimate partner violence. Exposure to a wider range of early trauma or adversity is linked with antisocial behaviour more generally but does not necessarily distinguish perpetrators or victims of intimate partner violence (Dube *et al*, 2002).

No single theory (or framework) sufficiently explains intimate partner violence, even where there is some empirical evidence supporting it. Although intimate partner violence occurs more often in contexts where there is support for male authority in the family and women have less access to economic security, it is not clear why some individuals are more likely to be violent under such conditions than others. Because types of intimate partner violence vary between couples, there are likely multiple causes for its occurrence, even if one accepts the central role of coercive control supported by patriarchal social structures. The field has moved from vociferous debate between competing theories towards an integrative multidimensional approach characterised by a social ecology model applied by Heise (1998) to aetiological and risk factors for perpetration and experience of intimate partner violence. Heise's model shown in Fig. 1.1 conceptualises the aetiology of intimate partner violence as a complex interplay between personal, social and situational factors, rather than as having a single cause.

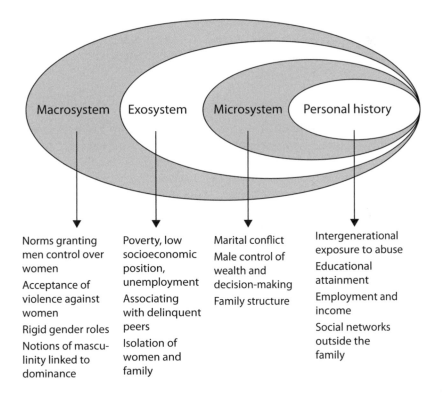

Fig. 1.1 An ecological framework of violence against women. Adapted from Heise (1998). © 1998 by SAGE. Reprinted with permission of SAGE Publications.

Physical health consequences of abuse

As well as measuring prevalence, the WHO multicountry study measured health status with a standardised questionnaire with the aim of assessing the extent to which physical and sexual violence were associated with adverse health outcomes (Ellsberg *et al*, 2008). The survey focused on general health and disabling symptoms. Pooled analysis of all 15 sites found significant associations between lifetime experiences of intimate partner violence and self-reported poor health and with specific health problems in the previous 4 weeks: difficulty walking, difficulty with daily activities, pain, memory loss, dizziness, and vaginal discharge. The increased risk varied by symptom, ranging from 50 to 80%. These significant associations were maintained in almost all of the sites. Between 19 and 55% of women who had ever been physically abused by their partner were ever injured.

The first burden of disease analysis of intimate partner violence was conducted in the Australian state of Victoria (Vos *et al*, 2006). It reported that intimate partner violence contributed 8% to the total disease burden in women aged 15 to 44 years and 3% in all women. Most strikingly, intimate partner violence was the leading contributor to death, disability and illness in women aged 15 to 44, being responsible for more of the disease burden than many well-known risk factors such as diabetes, high blood pressure, smoking and obesity. Poor mental health contributed 73% and substance misuse 22% to the disease burden attributed to intimate partner violence.

Reproductive health

Reproductive health problems have been the most extensively studied physical health consequences of intimate partner violence. In a systematic assessment of reviews up until 2008 (Feder *et al*, 2009), we found five reporting reproductive health effects. Here we summarise the findings of the more comprehensive reviews.

In a review of 14 published case–control and cohort studies, Murphy and colleagues (Murphy *et al*, 2001) meta-analysed the association between abuse during pregnancy and low birth weight in the child, finding a pooled odds ratio of 1.4 for a low-birth-weight baby in women who reported physical, sexual or emotional abuse during pregnancy, compared with women who were not abused. Boy & Salihu (2004) analysed 30 peer-reviewed studies on the impact of partner violence on pregnancy outcomes. Of the six studies focusing on maternal mortality, one case–control death review found that a woman abused during pregnancy was three times more likely to be killed by a partner. The remaining five studies on maternal mortality were based on death reviews and all noted that the majority of homicides were the result of partner violence. Similarly, the UK Confidential Enquiry into Maternal Deaths has consistently found a significant proportion of maternal deaths to be caused by homicide by a partner (Lewis, 2011).

Twenty-three studies looked at partner violence and pregnancy outcomes. Three cohort studies found no significant differences between women who were abused when pregnant and women who were not, seven studies reported mixed results, and the remaining thirteen found significant differences between the outcomes in these two groups. Six of the seven studies with mixed results reported a variety of negative behaviours during pregnancy in women who were abused, particularly substance misuse, and complications. Women who were abused were three times more likely to have kidney infections and were one-and-a-half times more likely to deliver by Caesarean section.

A review of nursing studies (including qualitative designs) on the relationship between partner violence and women's reproductive health published after 1995 was conducted by Campbell and colleagues (Campbell *et al*, 2000). Two studies examined the effects of forced sex on women's health. One study found that women who were sexually assaulted had significantly more gynaecological problems than those who were not sexually assaulted ($P=0.026$). The second study found that women who were sexually and physically abused had more physical health symptoms than those who were only sexually abused. One study investigated the association between abuse and risk of sexually transmitted infections, and found that the rate among the abused, assaulted and raped women was significantly higher than in those who were not. One study examined records from 389 victims of sexual assault, 71% of whom knew the perpetrator; it found that more than three-quarters of those resuming sexual activities reported sexual difficulties and 17.1% reported gynaecological pain, but almost all of them had normal general physical (98%) and gynaecological (95%) examinations.

Acute injury

Injuries are the most obvious manifestation of intimate partner violence; a clinician should have increased suspicion for intimate partner violence if the presenting history of injuries is not consistent with the physical examination, and when there is a delay in seeking medical care for injuries. Patients exposed to physical violence may present with injuries that vary from minor abrasions to life-threatening trauma. While there can be overlap between injuries resulting from intimate partner violence and injuries from other causes, the former typically involve trauma to the head, face and neck, with a meta-analysis of seven studies reporting an odds ratio of 24 for intimate partner violence in women with these injuries compared with women presenting with injuries at other sites (Wu *et al*, 2010). Multiple facial injuries are suggestive of intimate partner violence rather than of other causes and those that are more specific for intimate partner violence include zygomatic complex fractures, orbital blow-out fractures and perforated tympanic membrane. Musculoskeletal injuries are considered the second most common type of injuries, including sprains, fractures and dislocations. Blunt-force trauma to the forearms should raise suspicion of intimate partner violence, as this can occur when trying to block being struck.

The most severe consequence of domestic violence is death; in England and Wales, two women a week are killed by a partner or ex-partner (Povey, 2004). Women are at a greatest risk of violence from their partners when they attempt to leave and for several months after. Homicides may also involve other members of the family: in 2010/2011, 38% of all homicides (of victims aged 16 or older) in the UK were domestic related, with the murder of a parent by a child being most prevalent after that committed by a partner or ex-partner (Osborne, 2012).

Chronic physical health conditions

There are no systematic reviews of the chronic physical health consequences of intimate partner violence other than those addressing gynaecological and obstetric sequelae, summarised earlier (pp. 10–11). In addition to the WHO study, there are many cross-sectional studies, usually with convenience samples, showing increased risk of gastrointestinal, neurological and musculoskeletal syndromes (summarised in Campbell *et al*, 2002) in women who have experienced intimate partner violence, although confounding is possible and may limit interpretation. A well-designed study of 1152 consecutive female patients in two US family practices (Coker *et al*, 2000) found that women who experienced intimate partner violence had a significantly increased risk of: disability preventing work (1.6), chronic neck or back pain (1.5), arthritis (1.5), hearing loss (2.0), angina (2.0), bladder and kidney infections (1.7), sexually transmitted infections (3.1), chronic pelvic pain (1.5), stomach ulcers (2.0), irritable bowel syndrome (3.7); this was after controlling for potential confounders such as age, race, insurance status (as a proxy of income) and childhood exposure to intimate partner violence.

Impact on children

Exposure to intimate partner violence during childhood and adolescence is found to increase the risk of negative health outcomes across the lifespan. Reviews indicate a moderate to strong association between children's exposure to intimate partner violence and internalising symptoms (e.g. anxiety, depression), externalising behaviours (e.g. aggression) and trauma symptoms (e.g. flashbacks) (English *et al*, 2003; Kitzmann *et al*, 2003; Wolfe *et al*, 2003; Evans *et al*, 2008). Children exposed to domestic violence are estimated to be 2 to 4 times more likely to exhibit clinically significant problems than children from homes where there is no violence (McDonald & Jouriles, 1991; Cummings & Davies, 1994; Holden, 1998). Links are also demonstrated between children's exposure to violence and conflict and social development, academic attainment, engagement in risky health behaviours (e.g. smoking, substance misuse, early initiation of sexual activity) and other physical health consequences (Kolbo *et al*, 1996; Kitzmann *et al*, 2003; Bair-Merrit *et al*, 2006), although a more recent evidence synthesis concluded that there remains some uncertainty as to the magnitude and consistency of detrimental effects on these domains of children's functioning, whereas evidence relating to children's emotional and behavioural development is less equivocal (Feder *et al*, 2009). Several studies suggest that boys and girls may be differently affected by exposure (Wolfe *et al*, 2003; Evans *et al*, 2008) and that exposure may have a greater impact on younger children (Sternberg *et al*, 2006); in general, however, evidence relating to the moderating role of age and gender is unclear (Herrenkol *et al*, 2008).

Despite the fact that exposure to intimate partner violence undoubtedly constitutes a significant stressor in children's lives, studies indicate considerable variation in children's reactions and adaptation following exposure to this risky family context (Hughes & Luke, 1998; Grych *et al*, 2000). Heterogeneity in children's adaptation may in part be explained by the presence or absence of other adversities in their lives. For example, children exposed to intimate partner violence are at increased risk of being directly maltreated or neglected (e.g. Appel & Holden, 1998), with some evidence to indicate higher rates of maladjustment among children experiencing this 'double whammy' compared with children who are exposed to violence but not maltreated or neglected themselves (Hughes *et al*, 1989; Grych *et al*, 2000; Wolfe *et al*, 2003). Children exposed to or experiencing domestic violence may also be subject to a range of other adversities such as poverty, parental mental ill health, substance misuse and antisocial behaviour (Fantuzzo, *et al*, 1997; Margolin & Gordis, 2000; Appleyard *et al*, 2005), which may compound the effect of exposure to violence. The more adversities a child is exposed to, the greater their risk of experiencing negative health outcomes (Appleyard *et al*, 2005).

Conclusions

Domestic violence is common and is associated with numerous adverse health consequences for both adult and child victims. Although differing conceptualisations of domestic violence have led to some inconsistent findings, there is clear evidence that domestic violence is more prevalent in women who attend healthcare services, and it is therefore a major public health problem.

The next chapter discusses the evidence on mental health consequences of domestic violence, before we discuss, in chapters 3 and 4, how the mental health professional can address domestic violence experienced by people presenting to mental health services.

References

Abraham, M. (1999) Sexual abuse in South Asian immigrant marriages. *Violence Against Women*, **5**, 591–618.

Abrams, K. M. & Robinson, G. E. (1998) Stalking. Part 1: An overview of the problem. *Canadian Journal of Psychiatry*, **43**, 473–476.

Alhabib, S., Nur, U. & Jones, R. (2010) Domestic violence against women: systematic review of prevalence studies. *Journal of Family Violence*, **25**, 369–382.

Appel, A. E. & Holden, G. W. (1998) The co-occurrence of spouse and physical child abuse: a review and appraisal. *Journal of Family Psychology*, **12**, 578–599.

Appleyard, K., Egeland, B., van Dulmen, M. H., *et al* (2005) When more is not better: the role of cumulative risk in child behavior outcomes. *Journal of Child Psychology and Psychiatry*, **46**, 235–245.

Archer, J. (2000) Sex differences in aggression between heterosexual partners: a meta-analytic review. *Psychological Bulletin*, **126**, 651–680.

Arias I. & Pape K. T. (1999) Psychological abuse: implications for adjustment and commitment to leave violent partners. *Violence and Victims*, **14**, 55–67.

AuCoin, K. (ed.) (2005) *Family Violence in Canada: A Statistical Profile 2005*. Canadian Centre for Justice Statistics.

Bacchus, L., Mezey, G. & Bewley S. (2006) A qualitative exploration of the nature of domestic violence in pregnancy. *Violence Against Women*, **12**, 588–604.

Bair-Merrit, M. H., Blackstone, M. & Feudtner, C. (2006) Physical health outcomes of childhood exposure to intimate partner violence: a systematic review. *Pediatrics*, **117**, 278–290.

Beeble, M. L., Bybee, D. & Sullivan, C. M. (2007) Abusive men's use of children to control their partners and ex-partners. *European Psychologist*, **12**, 54–61.

Bonomi, A. E., Anderson, M. L., Rivara, F. P., *et al* (2009) Health care utilization and costs associated with physical and nonphysical-only intimate partner violence. *Health Services Research*, **44**, 1052–1067.

Boy, A. & Salihu, H. M. (2004) Intimate partner violence and birth outcomes: a systematic review. *International Journal of Fertility*, **49**, 159–163.

Brennan, S. (2011) Section 1: Self-reported spousal violence, 2009. In *Family Violence in Canada: A Statistical Profile*, pp. 8–19. Canadian Centre for Justice Statistics.

Britton, A. (2012) Intimate violence: 2010/11 BCS. In *Homicides, Firearm Offences and Intimate Violence 2010/2011: Supplementary Volume 2 to Crime in England and Wales 2010/11* (eds K. Smith, S. Osborne, I. Lau, *et al*), pp. 83–115. Home Office Statistical Bulletin.

Burke, P. J., Stets, J. E. & Pirog-Good, M. A. (1989) Gender identity, self-esteem and physical and sexual abuse in dating relationships. In *Violence in Dating Relationships* (eds M. A. Pirog-Good & J. E. Stets), pp. 72–93. Praeger.

Campbell, J. C., Woods, A. B., Laughon Choauf, K., *et al* (2000) Reproductive health consequences of intimate partner violence: a nursing research review. *Clinical Nursing Research*, **9**, 217–237.

Campbell, J., Jones, A.S., Dienemann, J., *et al* (2002) Intimate partner violence and physical health consequences. *Archives of Internal Medicine*, **162**, 1157–1163.

Carbone-Lopez, K., Kruttschnitt, C. & Macmillan, R. (2006) Patterns of intimate partner violence and their associations with physical health, psychological distress, and substance use. *Public Health Reports*, **121**, 382–392.

Catalano, S. M. (2012) *Intimate Partner Violence 1993–2010*. Bureau of Justice Statistics.

Coker, A. L., Smith, P. H., Bethea, L., *et al* (2000) Physical health consequences of physical and psychological intimate partner violence. *Archives of Family Medicine*, **9**, 1–7.

Cummings, E. M. & Davies, P. T. (1994) *Children and Marital Conflict: The Impact of Family Dispute and Resolution*. Guilford Press.

Desai, S. & Saltzman, L. (2001) Measurement issues for violence against women. In *Sourcebook on Violence Against Women* (eds C. Renzetti, J. Edleson & R. Bergen), pp. 35–52. Sage.

Dobash, R. P. & Dobash, R. E. (1979) *Violence Against Wives: A Case Against the Patriarchy*. Free Press.

Dobash, R. P., Dobash, E., Wilson, M., *et al* (1992) The myth of sexual symmetry in marital violence. *Social Problems*, **39**, 71–91.

Dube, S. R., Anda, R. F., Felitti, V. J., *et al* (2002) Exposure to abuse, neglect, and household dysfunction among adults who witnessed intimate partner violence as children: implications for health and social services. *Violence and Victims*, **17**, 3–17.

Dutton, M. A. & Goodman, L. A. (2005) Coercion in intimate partner violence: toward a new conceptualization. *Sex Roles*, **52**, 743–756.

Ellsberg, M., Jansen, H. A., Heise, L., *et al* (2008) Intimate partner violence and women's physical and mental health in the WHO multi-country study on women's health and domestic violence: an observational study. *Lancet*, **371**, 1165–1172.

English, D. J., Marshall, D. B. & Stewart, A. J. (2003) Effects of family violence on child behaviour and health during early childhood. *Journal of Family Violence*, **18**, 43–57.

Evans, S. E., Davies, C. & DiLillo, D. (2008) Exposure to domestic violence: a meta-analysis of child and adolescent outcomes. *Aggression and Violent Behavior*, **13**, 131–140.

Fantuzzo, J. W., Boruch, R., Beriana, A., *et al* (1997) Domestic violence and children: prevalence and risk in five major cities. *Journal of the American Academy of Child and Adolescent Psychiatry*, **36**, 116–122.

Feder, G., Ramsay, J., Dunne, D., *et al* (2009) How far does screening women for domestic (partner) violence in different health-care settings meet criteria for a screening programme? Systematic reviews of nine UK National Screening Committee criteria. *Health Technology Assessment*, **13**, iii–xiii.

Follingstad, D. R., Rutledge, L. L., Berg, B. J., *et al* (1990) The role of emotional abuse in physically abusive relationships. *Journal of Family Violence*, **5**, 107–120.

Garcia-Moreno, C., Jansen, H., Ellsberg, M., *et al* (2006) Prevalence of intimate partner violence: findings from the WHO multi-country study on women's health and domestic violence. *Lancet*, **368**, 1260–1269.

Geffner, R., Rosenbaum, A. & Hughes, H. (1988) Research issues concerning family violence. In *Handbook of Family Violence* (eds V. B. Van Hasselt, R. L. Morrison, A. S. Bellack, *et al*), pp. 457–481. Plenum Press.

Gordon, J. S. (2000) Definitional issues in violence against women. *Violence Against Women*, **6**, 747–783.

Graham-Kevan, N. & Archer, J. (2003a) Physical aggression and control in heterosexual relationships: the effect of sampling procedure. *Violence and Victims*, **18**, 181–198.

Graham-Kevan, N. & Archer, J. (2003b) Patriarchal terrorism and common couple violence: a test of Johnson's predictions in four British samples. *Journal of Interpersonal Violence*, **18**, 1247–1270.

Grych, J. H., Jouriles, E. N., Swank, P. R., *et al* (2000) Patterns of adjustment among children of battered women. *Journal of Consulting and Clinical Psychology*, **68**, 84–94.

Hall, P. & Innes, J. (2010) Violent and sexual crime. In *Crime in England and Wales 2009/10: Findings from the British Crime Survey and Police Recorded Crime* (3rd edn) (eds J. Flatley, C. Kershaw, K. Smith, *et al*), pp. 45–60. Home Office Statistical Bulletin.

Hegarty, K. (2006) What is intimate partner abuse and how common is it? In *Intimate Partner Abuse and Health Professionals: New Approaches to Domestic Violence* (eds G. Roberts, K. Hegarty & G. Feder), pp. 19–40. Elsevier.

Heise, L. L. (1998) Violence against women: an integrated, ecological framework. *Violence Against Women*, **4**, 262–290.

Heise, L., Ellsberg, M. & Gottemoeller, M. (1999) Population Reports: Ending violence against women. *Issues in World Health*, Series L, Number 11. The Johns Hopkins University School of Public Health (http://www.vawnet.org/Assoc_Files_VAWnet/PopulationReports.pdf).

Herrenkol, T. I., Sousa, C., Tajima, E. A., *et al* (2008) Intersection of child abuse and children's exposure to domestic violence. *Trauma, Violence and Abuse*, **9**, 84–99.

Holden, G. W. (1998) Introduction: the development of research into another consequence of family violence. In *Children Exposed to Marital Violence: Theory, Research and Applied Issues* (eds G. W. Holden, R. Geffner & E. N. Jouriles), pp. 1–20. American Psychological Association.

Home Office (2012) Domestic violence. Home Office (http://www.homeoffice.gov.uk/crime/violence-against-women-girls/domestic-violence/).

Hughes, H. M. & Luke, D. A. (1998) Heterogeneity in adjustment among children of battered women. In *Children Exposed to Marital Violence: Theory, Research and Applied Issues* (eds G. W. Holden, R. Geffner & E. N. Jouriles), pp. 185–221. American Psychological Association.

Hughes, H. M., Parkinson, D. & Vargo, M. (1989) Witnessing spouse abuse and experiencing physical abuse: a 'double whammy'? *Journal of Family Violence*, **4**, 197–209.

Johnson, M. P. (1995) Patriarchal terrorism and common couple violence: two forms of violence against women. *Journal of Marriage and the Family*, **57**, 283–294.

Johnson, M. P. (2006) Conflict and control. *Violence Against Women*, **12**, 1003–1018.

Kamphuis, J. H. & Emmelkamp, P. M. (2001) Traumatic distress among support-seeking female victims of stalking. *American Journal of Psychiatry*, **158**, 795–798.

Kitzmann, K. M., Gaylord, N. K., Holt, A. R., *et al* (2003) Child witnesses to domestic violence: a meta-analytic review. *Journal of Consulting and Clinical Psychology*, **71**, 339–352.

Kolbo, J. R., Blakely, E. H. & Engelman, D. (1996) Children who witness domestic violence: a review of empirical literature. *Journal of Interpersonal Violence*, **11**, 281–293.

Krug, E., Dahlberg, L. L., Mercy, J. A., *et al* (eds) (2002a) Violence by intimate partners. In *World Report on Violence and Health*, pp. 87–122. World Health Organization.

Krug, E., Dahlberg, L. L., Mercy, J. A., *et al* (eds) (2002b) *World Report on Violence and Health*. World Health Organization.

Lewis, G. (2011) Saving Mothers' Lives: reviewing maternal deaths to make motherhood safer: 2006–2008. The Eighth Report of the Confidential Enquiries into Maternal Deaths in the United Kingdom. *BJOG: An International Journal of Obstetrics and Gynaecology*, **118** (suppl. 1), 1–203.

Mahoney, P., Williams, L. M. & West, C. M. (2001) Violence against women by intimate relationship partners. In *Sourcebook on Violence against Women* (eds C. Renzetti, J. Edleson & R. K. Bergen), pp. 143–178. Sage.

Margolin, G. & Gordis, E. B. (2000) The effects of family and community violence on children. *Annual Review of Psychology*, **51**, 445–479.

Marshall, L. L. (1996) Psychological abuse of women: six distinct clusters. *Journal of Family Violence*, **11**, 379–409.

McCloskey, L. A. (2001) The 'Medea complex' among men: the instrumental abuse of children to injure wives. *Violence and Victims*, **16**, 19–37.

McDonald, R. & Jouriles, E. N. (1991) Marital aggression and child behaviour problems: research findings, mechanisms, and intervention strategies. *Behavior Therapist*, **14**, 189–192.

Mirlees-Black, C. (1999) *Domestic Violence: Findings From the British Crime Survey Self Completion Questionnaire*. Home Office.

Mitchell, C. & Vanya, M. (2009) Explanatory frameworks of intimate partner violence. In *Intimate Partner Violence: A Health-Based Perspective* (eds C. Mitchell & D. Anglin), pp. 39–52. Oxford University Press.

Murphy, C. M. & Hoover, S. A. (1999) Measuring emotional abuse in dating relationships as a multifactorial construct. *Violence and Victims*, **14**, 39–53.

Murphy, C. C., Schei, B., Myhr, T. L., *et al* (2001) Abuse: a risk factor for low birth weight? A systematic review and meta-analysis. *Canadian Medical Association Journal*, **164**, 1567–1572.

Nicolaidis, C. & Paranjape, A. (2009) Defining intimate partner violence: controversies and implications. In *Intimate Partner Violence: A Health-Based Perspective* (eds C. Mitchell & D. Anglin), pp. 19–38. Oxford University Press.

Okun, L. (1986) *Woman Abuse: Facts Replacing Myths*. SUNY Press.

O'Leary, K. D. (1999) Psychological abuse: a variable deserving critical attention in domestic violence. *Violence and Victims*, **14**, 3–23.

Osborne, S. (2012) Homicide. In *Homicides, Firearm Offences and Intimate Violence 2010/2011: Supplementary Volume 2 to Crime in England and Wales 2010/11* (eds K. Smith, S. Osborne, I. Lau, *et al*), pp. 15–29. Home Office Statistical Bulletin.

Pickett, K. & Wilkinson, R. (2009) *The Spirit Level: Why Equality is Better for Everyone*. Allen Lane.

Povey, D. (ed.) *(2004) Crime in England and Wales 2002/3: Supplementary Volume 1 – Homicide and Gun Crime*. Home Office Statistical Bulletin.

Rodgers, K. (1994) Wife assault: the findings of a national survey. *Juristat*, **14**, 1–21.

Saltzman, L. E., Fanslow, J. L., McMahon, P. M., *et al* (2002) *Intimate Partner Violence Surveillance: Uniform Definitions and Recommended Data Elements (version 1.0)*. Centers for Disease Control and Prevention, National Center for Injury Prevention and Control.

Sinha, M. (2012) Family violence in Canada: a statistical profile, 2010. *Statistics Canada catalogue*, no. 85–002–X.

Smith, K., Coleman, K., Eder, S., *et al* (2011) *Homicides, Firearm Offences and Intimate Violence 2009/10 (Supplementary Volume 2 to Crime in England and Wales 2009/10 2nd Edition)*. Home Office Statistical Bulletin.

Stark, E. (2009) *Coercive Control: How Men Entrap Women in Personal Life*. Oxford University Press.

Stark, E. & Buzawa, E. (eds) (2009) *Violence Against Women in Families and Relationships: Making and Breaking Connections. Volume II: Family Pieces*. Praeger Publishers.

Sternberg, K. J., Lamb, M. E., Gutterman, E., *et al* (2006) Adolescents' perceptions of attachments to their mothers and fathers in families with histories of domestic violence: a longitudinal perspective. *Child Abuse and Neglect*, **29**, 853–869.

Straus, M. (1986) Domestic violence and homicide antecedents. *Bulletin of the New York Academy of Medicine*, **62**, 446–465.

Straus, M. A. (1990) The Conflict Tactics Scale and its critics: an evaluation and new data on validity and reliability in physical violence. In *American Families: Risk Factors and Adaptations to Violence in 8145 Families* (eds M. A. Straus & R. J. Gelles). Transaction Publishers.

Straus, M. A. (1997) Physical assaults by women partners: a major social problem. In *Women, Men and Gender: Ongoing Debates* (ed. M. R. Walsh), pp. 210–221. Yale University Press.

Tjaden, P. & Thoennes, N. (1998) *Stalking in America: Findings from the National Violence Against Women Survey*. U.S. Department of Justice.

Vos, T., Astbury, J., Piers, L. S., *et al* (2006) Measuring the impact of intimate partner violence on the health of women in Victoria, Australia. *Bulletin of the World Health Organization*, **84**, 739–744.

Walby, S. (2009) *The Cost of Domestic Violence: Up-Date 2009*. Lancaster University.

Walby, S. & Myhill, A. (2001) Comparing the methodology of the new national surveys of violence against women. *British Journal of Criminology*, **41**, 502–522.

Walby, S. & Allen, J. (2004) *Domestic Violence, Sexual Assault and Stalking: Findings from the British Crime Survey*. Home Office Research Study 276. Home Office.

Waltermaurer, E. (2005) Measuring intimate partner violence: you may only get what you ask for. *Journal of Interpersonal Violence*, **20**, 501–506.

Weis, J. (1989) Family violence research methodology and design. In *Family Violence* (eds L. Ohlin & M. Tonry), pp. 117–162. University of Chicago Press.

Wolfe, D. A. & Jaffe, P. G. (1999) Emerging strategies in the prevention of domestic violence. *Future Child*, **9**, 133–144.

Wolfe, D. A., Crooks, C. V., Lee, V., *et al* (2003) The effects of children's exposure to domestic violence: a meta analysis and critique. *Clinical Child and Family Psychology Review*, **6**, 171–187.

Wu, V., Huff, H. & Bhandari, M. (2010) Pattern of physical injury associated with intimate partner violence in women presenting to the emergency department: a systematic review and meta-analysis. *Trauma, Violence and Abuse*, **11**, 71–82.

CHAPTER 2

Domestic violence and mental health

Kylee Trevillion, Siân Oram and Louise M. Howard

Domestic violence has been shown to be associated with a range of mental health problems, including depression, post-traumatic stress disorder (PTSD), suicidal ideation, substance misuse, functional symptoms, and the exacerbation of psychotic symptoms (Golding, 1999; Campbell, 2002; Neria *et al*, 2005; Trevillion *et al*, 2012). In this chapter we review literature on the prevalence of domestic violence among men and women with mental disorders and present evidence that suggests a bi-directional causal relationship between domestic violence and mental disorders. We focus largely on intimate partner violence among women, but where data are available we present findings on domestic violence perpetrated by other family members and violence among men.

The prevalence of domestic violence in people with mental disorders

Community-based and non-psychiatric healthcare surveys

A recent review of the international literature found that there is a high prevalence of intimate partner violence among men and women across all diagnostic categories of mental disorder (Trevillion *et al*, 2012). The median prevalence of lifetime intimate partner violence among women was reported as 45.8% among those with depressive disorders, 27.6% among those with anxiety disorders and 61% among those with PTSD. In relation to men, two high-quality studies reported a prevalence of lifetime intimate partner violence among men with depressive disorders (5.3% and 31.3%) and men with anxiety disorders (7.4% and 27%). One high-quality study also reported a prevalence of 7.3% for lifetime intimate partner violence among men with PTSD. The review found that there is a higher likelihood of experiencing adult lifetime partner violence among women with depressive disorders (odds ratio (OR)=2.77), anxiety disorders (OR=4.08) and PTSD (OR=7.34), compared with women without mental disorders. Although it was not possible to calculate pooled odds for other mental disorders and for domestic violence among men, the reviewers found that individual studies reported increased odds of domestic violence for men and women across all diagnostic categories, including psychosis, with a higher prevalence reported for women.

Smaller studies, conducted in healthcare settings or with community samples, also contribute to knowledge in this area. For example, a study of 126 consecutive admissions to a French emergency care service examined domestic violence by an intimate partner or family member and reported a lifetime prevalence of 42.9% among men and women with depression (Lejoyeux et al, 2002). The majority of research, however, has focused particularly on the prevalence of intimate partner violence among women with depressive, anxiety and post-traumatic stress disorders. The majority of such studies have been conducted in the USA (Cascardi et al, 1995; Tolman & Rosen, 2001; Tuten et al, 2004; Chang et al, 2009; Cerulli et al, 2011) and other high-income countries, but a small number report on the prevalence of intimate partner violence among women with mental disorder in low-income countries. This evidence base makes it clear that intimate partner violence is a significant global public health problem which is consistently associated with an increased risk of mental disorders. A community-based survey conducted in Ethiopia, for example, found a prevalence of 71.9% for physical violence and a prevalence of 62.5% for sexual violence among women with depression (Deyessa et al, 2009). In Pakistan, a study of female primary care users found that 89.2% of women with depression and 89.5% of women with PTSD reported physical and psychological violence (Ayub et al, 2009), and a study of women attending gynaecology clinics with vaginal discharge found verbal and physical abuse was significantly greater among women with common mental disorders than among women without disorders (Khan et al, 2012).

Less evidence is available on the prevalence of intimate partner violence among people with psychotic disorders: in three studies among women with schizophrenia and non-affective psychosis the prevalence ranged from 41.7 to 83.3% (Danielson et al, 1998; Wong & Phillips, 2009; Friedman et al, 2011). Each of these study samples, however, included fewer than 25 women.

Psychiatric surveys that examine the relationship between mental disorders and violence victimisation (i.e. encompassing physical, sexual and emotional abuse regardless of the relationship between victim and abuser) also indicate that people with mental disorders are up to 11 times more likely to experience recent violence than the general population (Walsh et al, 2003; Teplin et al, 2005; Choe et al, 2008). People with mental disorders are also more likely to report recent violence than people with other disabilities (i.e. non-specific impairments and intellectual disability) (Hughes et al, 2012). A recent meta-analysis (Hughes et al, 2012) reported an increased risk of violence among men and women with mental disorders

19

(OR 3.86) compared with controls, although substantial heterogeneity was observed between risk estimates across studies. Psychiatric victimisation studies, however, rarely provide information about specific types and contexts of abuse (Maniglio, 2009), even if this information has been collected.

As people with mental disorders are more likely to be victims of violence in general, it is likely that those at risk of domestic violence may be at increased risk of suffering other forms of non-domestic violence. However, the hidden nature of domestic violence and the intimate relationship between the abuser and victim means that the violence is often more frequent and severe than other forms of abuse (Kropp *et al*, 2005).

Psychiatric healthcare surveys

A systematic review on the prevalence of domestic violence across psychiatric settings worldwide identified a median prevalence of lifetime intimate partner violence as 31.7% among female in-patients, 33% among female out-patients and 31.6% among males across mixed psychiatric settings (Oram *et al*, 2013). Most of the studies were, however, conducted with small numbers of service users who were recruited through convenience sampling. None of the studies identified in the review included a direct comparison with a general population, with those facing similar levels of socioeconomic deprivation or other clinical groups, making it difficult to draw conclusions on the extent to which mental health service users are at greater risk of domestic violence.

Few studies have examined the prevalence of domestic violence by non-intimate family members. A US study of 66 consecutive female admissions to a psychiatric in-patient service reported a lifetime prevalence (≥ 16 years of age) of 9.1% for physical violence by a father and 6.1% for physical violence by a brother (Bryer *et al*, 1987). A Swedish study conducted a comprehensive assessment of the prevalence of lifetime domestic violence among mixed psychiatric settings and attempted to survey, over the course of 1 week, all adult female users of psychiatric in-patient and out-patient services (Bengtsson-Tops *et al*, 2005). Self-administered questionnaires were completed by 1382 women, 25.6% of whom reported violence by a current partner, 23.1% by a previous partner and 11.1% by family members (experienced after 16 years of age).

In the UK, a study of female community mental health service users in south London found that 60% had experienced lifetime physical intimate partner violence and 40% of women reported injuries, with 15% reporting abuse in the previous year (Morgan *et al*, 2010). It is not yet clear to what extent there exist gender differences in the prevalence of domestic violence victimisation among people with severe mental illness but illnesses such as schizophrenia may increase the risk of becoming a victim for men as well as women.

The relationship between domestic violence and mental disorder

Multiple studies, conducted across a variety of countries and in a range of settings, suggest there is a high prevalence of intimate partner violence among women with mental disorder, and both men and women who are victims of intimate partner violence are at increased risk of experiencing mental disorders. This does not appear to be specific to certain disorders; studies (Golding, 1999; Campbell, 2007; Golinelli *et al*, 2009; Trevillion *et al*, 2012) have found associations with:

- depression
- anxiety disorders including post-traumatic stress disorder (PTSD)
- eating disorders
- bipolar disorders (I and II)
- psychotic disorders
- antenatal and postnatal mental disorders, and
- alcohol and substance misuse.

Research also suggests that there is a causal association between domestic violence and mental disorder. A systematic review found, for example, that the severity and duration of physical intimate partner violence is associated with the frequency and severity of depression, and rates of depression decrease as time since the cessation of violence increases (Golding, 1999). A review which examined PTSD among victims of domestic violence similarly reported that the extent, severity and type of abuse were associated with the intensity of post-traumatic stress symptoms (Jones *et al*, 2001). Although women's experiences of physical, psychological and sexual abuse often overlap (Krug *et al*, 2002; Watts & Zimmerman, 2002), studies suggest that women who experience more than one form of abuse, or who are re-victimised, are at increased risk of mental disorder and comorbidity (McFarlane *et al*, 1998; Roberts *et al*, 1998; Jones *et al*, 2001; Romito *et al*, 2005; Tiwari *et al*, 2005; World Health Organization, 2013).

Mental disorder as a risk factor for domestic violence

The Dunedin Multidisciplinary Health and Development Study in New Zealand, a representative birth cohort study, found that psychiatric disorder can increase vulnerability to domestic violence (women who experienced abuse between the ages of 24 and 26 had reported significantly higher rates of major depression and substance misuse at age 18 than women in the same age group who had not been subjected to violence) and domestic violence was associated with an increased risk of psychiatric disorder among women at age 26 even after controlling for a history of mental disorder (Ehrensaft *et al*, 2006). Data from the National Survey of Families and Households, a nationally representative US cohort, similarly suggest that women who experience domestic violence are more likely to report depressive symptoms after 5 years of follow-up (Zlotnick *et al*, 2006), whereas a pregnancy cohort study reported that antenatal violence was associated with postnatal depression (Ludermir *et al*, 2010).

There is also evidence that women with pre-existing mental disorders may experience an exacerbation of symptoms if they are victims of domestic violence (Neria *et al*, 2005). Mental disorder may increase vulnerability to domestic violence by increasing the likelihood of women being in unsafe relationships and environments (McHugo *et al*, 2005) and increase their vulnerability to violent victimisation (Briere & Jordan, 2004; World Health Organization & London School of Hygiene and Tropical Medicine, 2010). Indeed, research suggests that men and women with severe mental illness face 12 times the risk of violent victimisation (of all types) compared with the general population (Teplin *et al*, 2005).

Potential pathways linking intimate partner violence and psychiatric disorder include:

(a) the association of intimate partner violence with other factors linked with mental health difficulties (e.g. impairments in social functioning, use of medication and poor living conditions or co-occurring substance misuse);
(b) previous physical and sexual abuse (including witnessing domestic violence as a child and previous intimate partner violence);
(c) trauma-induced intrusive thoughts (leading to the modification of coping styles and subsequent maladaptive choices that bring about violence-related trauma).

Evidence that domestic violence is a causal factor in the development of mental disorder further underlines the importance of domestic violence as a public health issue. The calculation of population attributable fractions (PAFs) is one way of quantifying the public health implications of domestic violence. Population attributable fractions represent the proportion of mental disorders that can be attributed to exposure to domestic violence, based on an assumption of causality. The domestic violence-related PAF for postnatal depression, for example, was recently estimated to be 10% in a Brazilian population (Ludermir *et al*, 2010). An Australian study estimated domestic violence-related PAFs for women aged 18–44 years at 21% for major depression and 17% for anxiety (Vos *et al*, 2006). Similar estimates were also found among women in a South African population (Norman *et al*, 2010). Such estimates suggest that reducing the prevalence of domestic violence could contribute to a substantial reduction in the burden of mental disorder and lower health service costs; in England and Wales alone it is estimated that direct medical and mental healthcare costs for domestic violence exceed £1730 million per annum (Walby, 2009).

Impact of domestic violence on mental disorders

As highlighted earlier, people with mental disorders are at increased risk of violent victimisation, which is shown to be associated with the onset, duration and recurrence of mental disorders (Brown *et al*, 1994). However, chronic traumatisation among victims of domestic violence has been shown to result in greater levels of psychiatric symptomatology (Herman, 1992), as is outlined below.

Pico-Alfonso *et al* (2006) compared three groups of women (non-abused, physically/psychologically abused and psychologically abused by their partners). They found that all the women who were subjected to physical violence also suffered from some form of psychological violence, with many also being sexually abused by their partners. The women exposed to physical/psychological and psychological abuse alone had a higher incidence and severity of depressive and anxiety symptoms, PTSD and thoughts of suicide than the control sample, with no differences between the two abused groups. Sexual violence was associated with a higher severity of depressive symptoms and a higher incidence of suicide attempts, whether the depressive symptoms were alone or comorbid with PTSD. State trait anxiety and thoughts of suicide were higher in abused women with depressive symptoms or comorbidity. Attempts at suicide were not, however, associated with specific symptomatology. This study, as do others (e.g. Jones *et al*, 2001; Coker *et al*, 2002; Romito *et al*, 2005), indicates that psychological violence can be as detrimental to mental health as physical violence. Perhaps surprisingly, exposure to psychological abuse can be more strongly and uniquely associated with PTSD symptoms than physical abuse (Taft *et al*, 2005).

The impact of domestic violence has been thought to have psychological parallels with the trauma of being taken hostage and subjected to torture (Dutton, 1992; Herman, 2001). Domestic abuse has been shown to have deleterious effects beyond other traumatic events. Research comparing Israeli women who had experienced domestic violence against women victimised by other traumatic events found that 52% of victims of domestic violence met the criteria for PTSD, and those reporting domestic violence experienced greater psychiatric symptomatology and suicide risk than those not reporting domestic violence (Sharhabani-Arzy *et al*, 2003).

Post-traumatic stress sequelae associated with domestic violence have undergone detailed examination in response to the complex presentation seen among victims exposed to extensive control and repeated assaults over a protracted period of time. Consequently, PTSD symptoms experienced by victims of domestic violence are seen to extend beyond the classic cluster of intrusive, avoidance and arousal symptoms to incorporate alterations in the victim's relationship to self, distorted relations with others and loss of sustaining beliefs, which characterises complex traumatic stress syndrome (Herman, 2001). Additional key features of this presentation include pervasive personality disturbances, including borderline personality

23

features (Pelcovitz *et al*, 1997). There is evidence to suggest that in some women alcohol and drug misuse is directly attributable to domestic abuse, as a manifestation of PTSD-avoidant dynamics (Campbell & Lewandowski, 1997; Campbell, 2007). Women who experience domestic violence are up to six times more likely to misuse or develop dependency on alcohol and drugs (Becker & Duffy, 2002; Golding, 1999).

Alongside managing psychiatric symptoms, victims of intimate partner violence are faced with multiple additional stressors associated with the violence, including (Jones *et al*, 2001; Rose *et al*, 2011):

- fear of further violence
- isolation and lack of social support
- mourning the loss of an intimate relationship
- concerns related to the welfare of their children
- concerns related to insecure immigration status
- fear of disruptions to family life/social networks/employment in the event of relocation
- fear of Social Services involvement and consequent child protection proceedings.

These factors also act as barriers to disclosure among victims of domestic violence when in contact with psychiatric services (Fig. 2.1, p. 25).

As will be outlined in Chapter 5, the chronic traumatisation experienced by victims of domestic violence highlights the need for trauma-based treatments, which are delivered in a context that addresses victims' current needs and does not impede on their ability to utilise key sources of support and to establish physical safety (Johnson & Zlotnick, 2010).

Conclusions

There is a strong association between domestic violence and mental disorder, with evidence of bi-directional causality. Mental health services, in both primary and secondary care, should therefore ensure that domestic violence is identified to reduce risk of further violence, improve safety and potentially improve mental health.

The next two chapters discuss how to identify and respond to mental health service users who are victims of domestic violence.

References

Ayub, M., Irfan, M., Nasr, T., *et al* (2009) Psychiatric morbidity and domestic violence: a survey of married women in Lahore. *Social Psychiatry and Psychiatric Epidemiology*, **44**, 953–960.

Becker, J. & Duffy, C. (2002) *Women Drug Users and Drugs Service Provision: Service Level Responses to Engagement and Retention (Briefing Paper)*. Home Office.

Bengtsson-Tops, A., Markstrom, U. & Lewin, B. (2005) The prevalence of abuse in Swedish female psychiatric users, the perpetrators and places where abuse occurred. *Nordic Journal of Psychiatry*, **59**, 504–510.

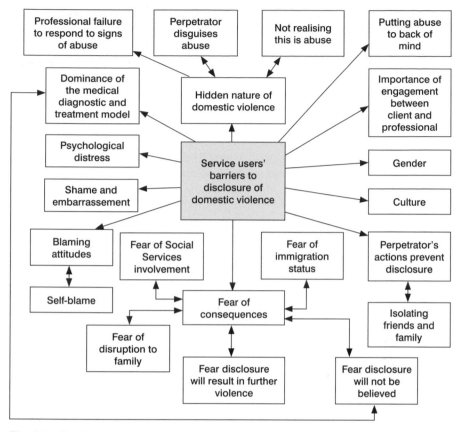

Fig. 2.1 Service users' barriers to disclosures of domestic violence (Source: Rose *et al*, 2011).

Briere, J. & Jordan, C. E. (2004) Violence against women: outcome complexity and implications for assessment and treatment. *Journal of Interpersonal Violence*, **19**, 1252–1276.

Brown, G. W., Harris, T. O., Hepworth, C., *et al* (1994) Clinical and psychosocial origins of chronic depressive episodes. II. A patient enquiry. *British Journal of Psychiatry*, **165**, 457–65.

Bryer, B. J., Nelson, A. B., Miller, B. J., *et al* (1987) Childhood sexual and physical abuse as factors in adult psychiatric illness. *American Journal of Psychiatry*, **144**, 1426–1430.

Campbell, J. C. (2002) Health consequences of intimate partner violence. *Lancet*, **359**, 1331–1336.

Campbell, J. C. (2007) *Assessing Dangerousness: Violence by Batterers and Child Abusers.* Springer.

Campbell, J. C. & Lewandowski, L. A. (1997) Mental and physical health effects of intimate partner violence on women and children. *Psychiatric Clinics of North America*, **20**, 1–23.

Cascardi, M., O'Leary, K., Lawrence, E. E., *et al* (1995) Characteristics of women physically abused by their spouses and who seek treatment regarding marital conflict. *Journal of Consulting and Clinical Psychology*, **63**, 616–623.

Cerulli, C., Talbot, N. L., Tang, W., *et al* (2011) Co-occurring intimate partner violence and mental health diagnoses in perinatal women. *Journal of Women's Health*, **20**, 1–7.

Chang, D. F., Shen, B. J. & Takeuchi, D. T. (2009) Prevalence and demographic correlates of intimate partner violence in Asian Americans. *International Journal of Law and Psychiatry*, **32**, 167–175.

Choe, J. Y., Teplin, L. A. & Abram, K. M. (2008) Perpetration of violence, violent victimization, and severe mental illness: balancing public health concerns. *Psychiatric Services*, **59**, 153–164.

Coker, A. L., Davis, K. E., Arias, I., *et al* (2002) Physical and mental health effects of intimate partner violence for men and women. *American Journal of Preventive Medicine*, **23**, 260–268.

Danielson, K. K., Moffitt, T. E., Caspi, A., *et al* (1998) Comorbidity between abuse of an adult and DSM-III-R mental disorders: evidence from an epidemiological study. *American Journal of Psychiatry*, **155**, 131–133.

Deyessa, N., Berhane, Y., Alem, A., *et al* (2009) Intimate partner violence and depression among women in rural Ethiopia: a cross-sectional study. *Clinical Practice and Epidemiology in Mental Health*, **5**, 8.

Dutton, M. A. (1992) *Empowering and Healing the Battered Woman: A Model for Assessment and Intervention*. Springer.

Ehrensaft, M. K., Moffitt, T. E. & Caspi, A. (2006) Is domestic violence followed by an increased risk of psychiatric disorders among women but not among men? A longitudinal cohort study. *American Journal of Psychiatry*, **163**, 885–892.

Friedman, S., Loue, S., Goldman Heaphy, E., *et al* (2011) Intimate partner violence victimization and perpetration by Puerto Rican women with severe mental illnesses. *Community Mental Health Journal*, **47**, 156–163.

Golding, M. J. (1999) Intimate partner violence as a risk factor for mental disorders: a meta-analysis. *Journal of Family Violence*, **14**, 99–132.

Golinelli, D., Longshore, D. & Wenzel, S. L. (2009) Substance use and intimate partner violence: clarifying the relevance of women's use and partners' use. *Journal of Behavioral Health Services & Research*, **36**, 199–211.

Herman, J. (1992) Complex PTSD: a syndrome in survivors of prolonged and repeated trauma. *Journal of Traumatic Stress*, **5**, 377–391.

Herman, J. (ed.) (2001) *Trauma and Recovery: From Domestic Abuse to Political Terror*. Rivers Oram/Pandora.

Hughes, K., Bellis, M. A., Jones, L., *et al* (2012) Prevalence and risk of violence against adults with disabilities: a systematic review and meta-analysis of observational studies. *Lancet*, **379**, 1621–1629.

Johnson, D. M. & Zlotnick, C. (2010) HOPE for battered women with PTSD in domestic violence shelters. *Professional Psychology: Research and Practice*, **40**, 234–241.

Jones, L., Hughes, M. & Unterstaller, U. (2001) Post traumatic stress disorder (PTSD) in victims of domestic violence: a review of the research. *Trauma, Violence and Abuse*, **2**, 99–119.

Khan, N., Kausar, R., Flach, C., *et al* (2012) Psychological and gynaecological morbidity in women presenting with vaginal discharge in Pakistan. *International Journal of Culture and Mental Health*, **5**, 169–181.

Kropp, P. R., Hart, S. D. & Belfrage, H. (2005) *The Brief Spousal Assault Form for the Evaluation of Risk (B-SAFER)*. Proactive Resolutions.

Krug, E., Mercy, J., Dahlberg, L., *et al* (2002) The World Report on Violence and Health. *Lancet*, **360**, 1083–1088.

Lejoyeux, M., Zillhardt, P., Chièze, F., *et al* (2002) Screening for domestic violence among patients admitted to a French emergency service. *European Psychiatry*, **17**, 479–483.

Ludermir, A., Lewis, G. & Valongueiro, S. (2010) Violence against women by their intimate partner during pregnancy and postnatal depression: a prospective cohort study. *Lancet*, **376**, 903–910.

Maniglio, R. (2009) Severe mental illness and criminal victimization: a systematic review. *Acta Psychiatrica Scandinavica*, **119**, 180–191.

McFarlane, J., Parker, B., Soeken, K., *et al* (1998) Safety behaviors of abused women after an intervention during pregnancy. *Journal of Obstetric, Gynecologic & Neonatal Nursing*, **27**, 64–69.

McHugo, G. J., Kammerer, N., Jackson, E. W., *et al* (2005) Women, co-occurring disorders, and violence study: evaluation design and study population. *Journal of Substance Abuse and Treatment*, **28**, 91–107.

Morgan, J. F., Zolese, G., McNulty, J., *et al* (2010) Domestic violence among female psychiatric patients: cross-sectional survey. *Psychiatrist*, **34**, 461–464.

Neria, Y., Bromet, E. J., Carlson, G. A., *et al* (2005) Assaultive trauma and illness course in psychotic bipolar disorder: findings from the Suffolk county mental health project. *Acta Psychiatrica Scandinavica*, **111**, 380–383.

Norman, R., Schneider, M., Bradshaw, D., *et al* (2010) Interpersonal violence: an important risk factor for disease and injury in South Africa. *Population Health Metrics*, **8**, 1–12.

Oram, S., Trevillion, K., Feder, G., *et al* (2013) Prevalence of experiences of domestic violence among psychiatric patients: systematic review. *British Journal of Psychiatry*, **202**, 94–99.

Pelcovitz, D., Van der Kolk, B., Roth, S., *et al* (1997) Development of a criteria set and a structured interview for disorders of extreme stress (SIDES). *Journal of Traumatic Stress*, **10**, 3–16.

Pico-Alfonso, M. A., Garcia-Linares, M., Celda-Navarro, N., *et al* (2006) The impact of physical, psychological, and sexual intimate male partner violence on women's mental health: depressive symptoms, posttraumatic stress disorder, state anxiety, and suicide. *Journal of Women's Health*, **15**, 599–611.

Roberts, G. L., Lawrence, J. M., Williams, G. M., *et al* (1998) The impact of domestic violence on women's mental health. *Australian and New Zealand Journal of Public Health*, **22**, 796–801.

Romito, P., Turan, J. M. & Marchi, M. D. (2005) The impact of current and past interpersonal violence on women's mental health. *Social Science and Medicine*, **60**, 1717–1728.

Rose, D., Trevillion, K., Woodall, A., *et al* (2011) Barriers and facilitators of disclosures of domestic violence by mental health service users: qualitative study. *British Journal of Psychiatry*, **198**, 189–194.

Sharhabani-Arzy, R., Amir, M., Kotler, M., *et al* (2003) The toll of domestic violence. *Journal of Interpersonal Violence*, **18**, 1335.

Taft, C. T., Murphy, C. M., King, L. A., *et al* (2005) Posttraumatic stress disorder symptomatology among partners of men in treatment for relationship abuse. *Journal of Abnormal Psychology*, **114**, 259–268.

Teplin, L. A., McClelland, G. M., Abram, K. M., *et al* (2005) Crime victimization in adults with severe mental illness – comparison with the national crime victimization survey. *Archives of General Psychiatry*, **62**, 911–921.

Tiwari, A., Leung, W. C., Leung, T. W., *et al* (2005) A randomised controlled trial of empowerment training for Chinese abused pregnant women in Hong Kong. *BJOG: An International Journal of Obstetrics and Gynaecology*, **112**, 1249–1256.

Tolman, R. M. & Rosen, D. (2001) Domestic violence in the lives of women receiving welfare – mental health, substance dependence, and economic well-being. *Violence against Women*, **7**, 141–158.

Trevillion, K., Oram, S., Feder, G., *et al* (2012) Experiences of domestic violence and mental disorders: a systematic review and meta-analysis. *PLoS ONE*, **7**, e51740.

Tuten, M., Jones, H. E., Tran, G., *et al* (2004) Partner violence impacts the psychosocial and psychiatric status of pregnant, drug-dependent women. *Addictive Behaviors*, **29**, 1029–1034.

Vos, T., Astbury, J., Piers, L. S., *et al* (2006) Measuring the impact of intimate partner violence on the health of women in Victoria, Australia. *Bulletin of the World Health Organization*, **84**, 739–744.

Walby, S. (2009) *The Cost of Domestic Violence: Up-date 2009*. Lancaster University.

Walsh, E., Moran, P., Scott, C., *et al* (2003) Prevalence of violent victimisation in severe mental illness. *British Journal of Psychiatry*, **183**, 233–238.

Watts, C. & Zimmerman, C. (2002) Violence against women: global scope and magnitude. *Lancet*, **359**, 1232–1237.

Wong, S. P. Y. & Phillips, M. R. (2009) Nonfatal suicidal behavior among Chinese women who have been physically abused by their male intimate partners. *Suicide and Life Threatening Behavior*, **39**, 648–658.

World Health Organization (2013) *Guideline Development Group on Policy and Clinical Practice Guidelines for Responding to Violence against Women (2011–2012)*. WHO (in press).

World Health Organization & London School of Hygiene and Tropical Medicine (2010) *Preventing Intimate Partner and Sexual Violence against Women: Taking Action and Generating Evidence*. WHO.

Zlotnick, C., Johnson, D. M. & Kohn, R. (2006) Intimate partner violence and long-term psychosocial functioning in a national sample of American women. *Journal of Interpersonal Violence*, **21**, 262–275.

CHAPTER 3

Identifying domestic violence experienced by mental health service users

Roxane Agnew-Davies

This chapter explores issues to be considered when identifying domestic violence. A 'best practice' approach has been taken to the advice given, based on evidence where available, with guidelines for health and mental health professionals supplementing the evidence base (e.g. Department of Health & Home Office, 2000; Department of Health, 2005, 2009; British Medical Association, 2007; Foreign & Commonwealth Office, 2007; Greater London Domestic Violence Project, 2008; Ethnic Alcohol Counselling in Hounslow (EACH), 2009).

Indicators of domestic violence

As discussed in previous chapters, people attending mental healthcare services are more likely than the general population to be victims of domestic violence and professionals therefore need to be aware of current and previous domestic violence their patients may be experiencing. In addition to physical and mental health symptoms there are other indicators of possible domestic violence which should alert healthcare professionals (Box 3.1, p. 30). These are likely to occur across all in-patient and out-patient settings as there is a high prevalence of both previous and recent domestic violence in all mental health service users (Oram et al, 2013). Evidence to date suggests that women are at greatest risk of domestic violence (Barnish, 2004) and most of this chapter therefore refers to women rather than men. However, similar principles apply to men suffering from domestic violence and of course they too deserve appropriate support.

Barriers to disclosure

Only 10–30% of recent violence is asked about and identified in clinical practice (Howard et al, 2010). There may be powerful barriers preventing disclosure, which include the stages of change in victims' understanding of their experiences. Disclosure can seem an insurmountable challenge in the context of intimidation by the perpetrator/perpetrators, pressure

Box 3.1 Potential indicators of possible domestic violence

1 Acute physical injuries following assault:
   - bruising and injuries (e.g. bilateral bruising, burns, bite marks; genital trauma; injuries to face, head, neck, chest)
   - breaks and fractures (e.g. broken bones, orbital fractures, lost teeth)
   - miscarriage, foetal trauma, abdominal trauma
   - injuries or bruises in various stages of healing
   - injury inconsistent with explanation offered.
2 Chronic health problems:
   - gynaecological problems (e.g. pelvic pain, vaginal bleeding, STIs)
   - HIV
   - heart and circulatory conditions
   - complaints of aches and pains (e.g. headaches; back pain)
   - gastrointestinal disorders (e.g. irritable bowel syndrome)
   - stress-related symptoms (e.g. dizziness, chronic headache).
3 Psychological indicators:
   - post-traumatic stress disorder (PTSD)
   - depression, including suicide attempts and self-harming behaviours
   - problematic substance use (including prescribed drugs and alcohol)
   - anxiety disorders
   - sleep problems
   - exacerbation of psychotic symptoms.
4 Indicators in the behaviour of the victim:
   - covering the body to hide marks (long sleeves, trousers or scarves)
   - attending late or often missing appointments
   - frequent visits with vague complaints or different symptoms
   - seeming anxious, fearful or passive (particularly in presence of others)
   - giving inconsistent explanations for injuries, being evasive or embarrassed
   - not wanting letters, visits or contact at home.
5 Possible indicators in the behaviour of partner/another person:
   - cancellation of appointments on patient's behalf
   - always attends, talking on behalf of patient or appearing overly protective
   - bullying or aggressive; critical, judgemental or insulting about patient
   - evasive or, conversely, adamant about the cause of injury
   - over-vehement denial of violence or minimises its severity
   - does not consult patient about their wishes, needs or feelings
   - disturbed behaviour of the children.

STIs, sexually transmitted infections
Based on Department of Health, 2009; Trevillion *et al*, 2010.

to remain in the relationship from the wider family or community and suffering consequent on the abuse. A perpetrator may have tried to enforce secrecy and silence by threats, shaming and humiliation. They may control medication and undermine the victim's credibility with her social network, including her fitness as a parent. The perpetrator may accompany her to appointments, presenting as a solicitous and concerned partner or family member, who by their presence effectively silences her, since she knows that any disclosure could be met by their denial in the short term and further abuse after they leave the building. He may have threatened her life, access to her children or her family.

For lesbian, bisexual, gay or transgender people, the perpetrator may have threatened to 'out' him or her and internalised social homophobia may compound feelings of guilt, shame and powerlessness. For people living with a disability or mental illness, the perpetrator may also be their primary carer and fears about what will happen and who will look after them if they tell a professional about abuse can act as major barriers to disclosure.

Specific dynamics of abuse experienced by women from Black and minority ethnic and refugee communities can include the involvement or collusion of multiple perpetrators in communities in which divorce brings disgrace to the family, compounding any threats of rejection, removal, kidnapping, separation from children and murder, and these can converge to increase victims' fears and prevent disclosure (EACH, 2009). Gypsy and traveller women can face similar community pressures to remain married, not to seek outside help and to solve problems within the extended family. Problems such as language barriers, illiteracy, poverty, insecure status and dependency converge to keep victims and children isolated and entrapped (Mullender et al, 2002).

Although there is great diversity among Black and minority ethnic and refugee victims, many have common experiences when help-seeking, including uncertainty about where to go; discrimination or negative reactions from agencies (the police, housing, benefits agencies) and health professionals; feelings of responsibility for protecting their family; doubts about not being believed; professionals' beliefs that certain types of abuse are part of 'the culture'; and insecure immigration status (Rai & Thiara, 1997; Gill, 2004; EACH, 2009).

Victims of violence face difficulties in a society in which stigma around domestic violence and mental illness is widespread. Zweig et al (2002) identified additional barriers for women who had concerns with substance misuse, mental illness and intellectual disabilities (Zweig et al, 2002). These are numerous and are listed in Box 3.2 (p. 32).

In summary, women dealing with substance misuse issues, mental health problems or intellectual disabilities face many barriers to accessing services or receiving adequate support from community-based service providers. The problems that many women victims of violence face, such as housing or social isolation, are compounded and complicated by the other issues in their lives. For example, it is more difficult to help women access employment when they are also struggling with active substance misuse.

As discussed briefly in Chapter 2, a qualitative study of community mental health service users in south London found that barriers to disclosure included fear of consequences, including fear of Social Services' involvement and consequent child protection proceedings; fear that disclosure would not be believed, and that disclosure would lead to further violence; the hidden nature of the violence; actions of the perpetrator; and feelings of shame (Rose et al, 2011). However, one major barrier to disclosure is not being

---

Box 3.2 Barriers to help for women with substance misuse, mental ill health and intellectual disability who experience abuse

- Abusers exploit the extra problems women experience as abuse strategies in their own right to control, humiliate, hurt or further disable them (e.g. supplying alcohol or drugs; withholding necessary care or assistance with basic daily living tasks; leading or leaving women in vulnerable positions).
- The community, including the criminal justice system and health professionals, is more likely to blame victims, question their credibility and take them less seriously.
- Service providers feel they lack training in dual issues.
- Few services simultaneously tackle multiple issues a woman is coping with.
- Recovery from abuse is difficult enough to deal with, but it is made more difficult when a woman also has to deal with more issues. Each issue makes the other issues harder to resolve.
- Women with multiple barriers may have more restricted ability to understand what is happening, as a function of their intellectual disability or trauma.
- Women are dependent on others, reluctant to disclose problems and prone to self-blame because of their problems (e.g. substance misuse).
- They have experiences of being excluded, rejected or treated badly.
- Women facing multiple barriers are more likely to cancel or drop out of, and are less likely to be offered, follow-up appointments by health professionals than other women.

---

asked about domestic violence by healthcare professionals (as discussed in the next section). Barriers to asking by professionals include lack of confidence, knowledge and competence, with anxieties about consequences of asking (Fig. 3.1, p. 33; Rose *et al*, 2011). These are addressed in the next section.

Why, when and how to ask about domestic violence

Why ask directly?

It is clear from several studies that routine clinical interview and clinical records reflect considerable underdetection by mental health professionals of violence experienced by service users (MacMillan *et al*, 2006; Howard *et al*, 2010). Research has also found that service users often do not disclose abuse in the absence of direct questioning from health professionals (Taket *et al*, 2003; Read *et al*, 2005; Bacchus *et al*, 2008; Rose *et al*, 2011). These findings are noteworthy because mental health service users may not have direct contact with any other services, may face barriers to accessing help and their symptoms may be treated without understanding the underlying cause. Studies in psychiatric services are consistent with studies in other healthcare settings in that implementation of routine enquiry in psychiatric settings increases detection rates (Howard *et al*, 2010).

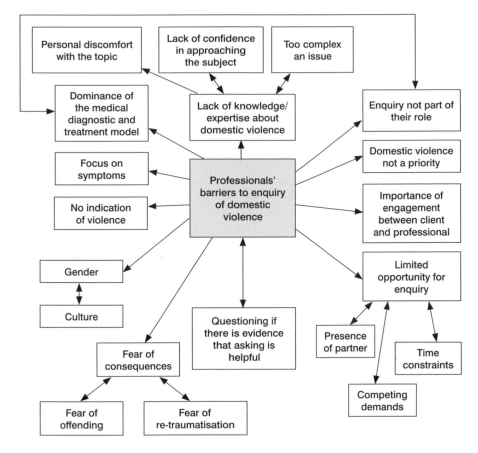

Fig. 3.1 Professionals' barriers to enquiry of domestic violence (Source: Rose *et al*, 2011).

In contrast to professional concerns, service users report feeling comfortable about being asked about domestic violence by health professionals (Feder *et al*, 2006; Rose *et al*, 2011; Trevillion *et al*, 2012). Enquiry is acceptable both to those service users who experience abuse and to those who do not (Rose *et al*, 2011). Similar views have been expressed by most women in contact with primary healthcare and maternity services (Ramsay *et al*, 2002; Bacchus *et al*, 2008).

Each mental health professional can play a pivotal role in suggesting that an experience of current or historic abuse is relevant to mental health assessment. When assessing for domestic violence, attention is focused on the aetiology of symptoms and concern shown about real, external danger, rather than treating the symptoms only. By asking about violence, the professional is giving important messages: you care about her safety; the problem is not too shameful to discuss; her distress is understandable; you hope the situation can change; abuse is wrong and not the responsibility of a victim; and they are not alone.

Policy in the UK is that clinical enquiry about domestic violence should form part of mental health assessments in psychiatric care (Department of Health, 2008, 2010). Asking about domestic abuse can:

- raise a patient's awareness about the ways domestic violence may have affected their mental health;
- identify more victims at risk;
- create an opportunity for frightened service users to disclose and decrease their feelings of isolation;
- provide victims with information about local and national services for people affected by domestic abuse;
- by preventative intervention, save the health service money and time;
- safeguard children and reduce long-term consequences of abuse on their mental health;
- play a part in holding perpetrators of abuse accountable.

Some professionals may feel that they cannot fully rely on service users' accounts of abuse. However, evidence suggests that psychiatric service users tend to under- rather than over-report victimisation experiences (Goodman *et al*, 1999).

When to ask

Talking about domestic violence needs to become part of the mental health professional's daily work. Current UK Department of Health policy is that following appropriate training for staff, exploration of violence and abuse should be routinely undertaken in all mental health assessments for men and women (Department of Health, 2008). There have been no randomised controlled trials to evaluate this policy of routine enquiry and training may not yet be available for all mental healthcare practitioners. Training and support is therefore needed to ensure that professionals feel confident to ask service users directly about domestic violence. Training and support should be commissioned from specialist domestic violence services, which is consistent with recommendations from the Department of Health Taskforce on the Health Aspects of Violence against Women and Children (2010).

An appropriate time to ask would be at initial assessment, when taking a social history or when asking about other factors that have a negative impact on mental health; at a care programme approach review; at change in admission status; and at change of keyworker. It may not always be possible to ask about domestic violence at initial assessments if the patient is acutely disturbed and agitated, but it is important not to forget to ensure that during the course of the ongoing assessment questions about domestic violence are asked. Disclosure is a process and many women will not disclose when first asked, so asking more than once over the course of a therapeutic relationship is essential.

Questions should not be asked in the presence of a partner or other family members. Good practice requires that mental health assessments must include seeing a patient alone at least once in a place where the conversation cannot be monitored or overheard, ensuring privacy and confidentiality. If an interpreter is needed, one who is unknown to the woman or her family must be used on this occasion.

Practitioners should be mindful of the indicators of domestic violence as illustrated in Box 3.1 (p. 30). As physical examination of a patient may be less likely in the mental health setting, professionals need to be alert to indicators in the behaviour of a patient and a person accompanying them.

How to ask

Creating the right environment

It is important that mental health services provide supportive environments so that victims have an opportunity to talk safely about domestic violence. Mental health professionals work in a variety of different contexts where the physical setting may be more or less comfortable or private. You should consider where to talk to each patient alone at least once, in a private area where you can talk one to one without being overheard.

Check whether there are posters on domestic violence services displayed in appropriate areas around your practice or department. Can victims get access safely and discreetly to information leaflets on domestic violence? Discreet areas include changing rooms or toilets. If general information is given to service users, this could be an opportunity to include leaflets on domestic violence services. Any information provided should reflect the diversity of the population, with provision in community languages, as well as addressing the specific needs of people with physical or intellectual disabilities. Research shows that domestic violence helplines and agencies are accessed directly by people who self-refer because they have seen posters or leaflets in healthcare agencies (Feder *et al*, 2009).

In a US study, women identified a number of qualities in health professionals that would facilitate disclosure of domestic violence (Rodriguez & Saba, 2006). These included creating a supportive environment, providing continued support, developing trust and reassurance of confidentiality. Women emphasised the need for health professionals to listen to their concerns and work at a pace with which they felt comfortable. The health professional's body language and facial expressions were identified as subtle but important means to show concern and develop trust. The approachability and confidence of staff can make a tremendous difference to whether or not a person feels comfortable and safe to talk about domestic violence.

Current evidence suggests that domestic violence enquiry is most likely to be effective if psychiatric professionals are trained to enhance confidence in their own ability to help people experiencing domestic violence and to improve their knowledge about domestic violence services (Howard *et al*, 2010). It depends on the clinical situation which type of assessment to carry out on a patient (initial screening or options for a more detailed assessment). Here, we provide the tools for a detailed assessment.

Asking the initial question

One single question about domestic violence, without follow-up, can improve disclosure rates by at least 10% (Barnish, 2004). Evidence from practice suggests that the majority of people do not mind being asked about their experiences of domestic violence when it is explained to them that the same enquiry is being made of all patients because domestic violence is widespread and often hidden (Harris *et al*, 2002; Bacchus *et al*, 2008), and when enquiry and disclosure are facilitated by a supportive and trusting relationship between patient and professional (Rose *et al*, 2011).

There is no one set list of questions that are best used when asking about domestic abuse. It is important that each professional develops a set of questions that suits their personal style. Initial comments or questions should attempt to put the patient at ease and help them to feel sufficiently safe and comfortable to discuss experiences if they wish, now or in the future. The aim is to have a supportive conversation and to indicate that information and help are available, rather than to force a disclosure.

A victim of domestic violence is likely to have been told it is her fault, that no one will believe her or that she will be judged negatively. Phrasing any question in terms of the abuser's behaviour can minimise the risk that the woman will feel to blame for the violence inflicted on her. For instance, on noticing an injury, the question 'Who hurt you?' is less likely to incur victim-blaming than 'How did you get that?'. Similarly, if a professional shares any reaction to the disclosure, it should be couched with reference to the abuser, for instance 'I am sad (or angry) that he did that to you', so that the woman does not feel herself to be a burden and so that she does not take responsibility for your reaction. However, denigrating the abuser should be avoided, and it is helpful to focus on the behaviour rather than the person.

UK guidelines recommend starting with a few open questions or a funnelling sentence before following up with specific questions about domestic violence (Bewley *et al*, 1997; British Medical Association, 2007; Social Care Institute for Excellence, 2011). Some examples of opening questions are given in Box 3.3 (p. 37).

Follow-up questions

If the patient says she has been frightened or hurt, you might ask more specific questions to explore her experiences of domestic violence. These can be grouped under the headings of physical abuse, sexual abuse or psychological abuse (including financial abuse and enforced social isolation), although each group overlaps and compounds the impact of others.

It is usually best to phrase questions in terms of the behaviour of the perpetrator rather than the effect on the victim. For example, you may ask, 'Has your partner or a relative ever:
- kicked, punched, pushed, grabbed or tried to choke or strangle you?'
- tried to hurt the children?'

Box 3.3   Possible opening questions for asking about abuse

- 'One in four women experience domestic violence at some time in their lives, and one in nine women have been hurt in the past 12 months. Has your partner or anyone else hurt or frightened you in any way?'
- 'Because domestic violence is so common, I ask everyone routinely. As an adult, have you been emotionally, physically or sexually abused by someone?'
- 'Over the past year, have you been hurt by someone, for example your partner, ex-partner or a family member?'
- 'How safe or afraid do you feel in your current relationship?'
- 'Is there anything that happens at home you are unhappy about?'
- 'How do arguments go in your house?'
- 'Who makes the decisions at home?'

If the patient has injuries:

- 'I've noticed a number of bruises/cuts/scars/marks. Who hurt you? What happened?'

It can help to convey that domestic violence is common and that you are familiar with dealing with the effects. For example, you could say:

- 'Many people I see with these sorts of injuries (or symptoms) have been experiencing domestic violence. Is a relative hurting you or threatening you?'

If the service user hesitates, you might say:

- 'I'm asking because I am concerned about all my patients' safety and to find out if you need information or support. I will not tell your family or partner about what you say.'

If the patient answers 'No', respect her response and choice. However, note any possible indicators of abuse such as non-verbal signs of hesitation, fear or a partner's behaviour that seems overly protective or controlling. Whether or not any signs associated with abuse are present, you might say:

- 'Because domestic violence happens to one in four women at some point, I let every woman know there is information and help available [specify where, such as in the waiting area or ladies' room] and that women who are at risk can call a free national domestic violence helpline. I also have a card with useful telephone numbers and contact details for domestic violence services that I give to people, if they are interested and it is safe for them to take it away.'

- threatened you or the children?'
- called you insulting names, made you feel small or insisted on what you wear?'
- broken or destroyed your property?'
- tried to stop you going to work/classes?'
- controlled the finances or denied you access to money?'
- got you to take drugs or alcohol when you haven't wanted to?'
- made you have sex in a way you did not want?'
- expected you to have sex when you didn't feel like it?'
- told you not to talk about problems outside the family or community?'

Box 3.4   Questions on sexual abuse

- Do you ever feel you have to go along with sex even though you don't want to?
- Have you felt forced into sex because of what your partner might do?
- Has anyone made you have sex or carried on when it was painful?
- Has anyone made you have oral or anal sex when you didn't want to?
- Has anyone used an object in a sexual way that you didn't like?
- Has anyone made you do things or perform sexual acts you didn't like?
- Has anyone refused safe sex or to use birth control?
- Has anyone made you have sex with another person?
- Has anyone talked about sex or done things in a way you didn't like?
- Have you been cut or stitched because of female genital mutilation or circumcision?

Box 3.5   Questions on physical abuse

- Has anyone shaken you or grabbed you roughly?
- Has anyone shoved you or made you fall?
- Has anyone slapped you or smacked you?
- Has anyone tried to hit you with something, used an object as a weapon?
- Has anyone punched you?
- Has anyone tried to choke you or put his hands round your throat?
- Has anyone pushed you against the wall or thrown you down?
- Has anyone pulled your hair?
- Has anyone burnt you or scalded you with something?
- Has anyone threatened you with a knife or gun?
- Has anyone hurt you while you were pregnant?

Box 3.6   Questions on psychological abuse

- Does anyone insult you, call you names or swear at you?
- Does anyone make it difficult for you to see friends/family or leave the house?
- Does anyone act in a jealous way or keep track of where you go?
- Does anyone put you down, embarrass you or criticise you?
- Does anyone undermine your independence or try to make you feel small?
- Does anyone make you feel as if you have to walk on eggshells or as if you do nothing right?
- Does anyone order you around like a servant?
- Does anyone blame you for things that are not your fault?
- Does anyone control money, make you ask for it or stop you earning?

Boxes 3.4–3.6 cover some questions that could be used to elicit disclosure of experiences of the different types of abuse.

The Power and Control Wheel (Fig. 3.2, p. 40) is a useful tool for exploring psychological abuse further with a patient. Simply providing a copy to the patient and asking whether they recognise any of these behaviours can help open up further discussion.

The Power and Control Wheel is a way of visually representing the tactics typically used by perpetrators of domestic violence. The wheel was created in 1982 by Ellen Pence, Coral McDonnell and Michael Paymar as part of a curriculum for a court-ordered programme for abusers (Pence & Paymar, 1986). It was developed out of the experiences of their violent partners attending support and educational groups in Duluth, Minnesota, USA and has been translated into 40 languages since then. The women were asked, 'What do you want taught in court-ordered groups for men who batter?'. Their answers highlighted the need to capture the complex reality of abuse and coercion. As the designers probed, women began to talk about the tactics their partners used to control them. Violence was commonplace. Less recognised but equally significant were other tactics of power, including control of money; the children; emotional and psychological put downs; undermining self-esteem and other social relationships; constant criticism of women's mothering; intimidation; and various forms of expressing male privilege or entitlement. Over the weeks the designers revised and adjusted the Wheel until the groups of women were satisfied that it captured their experience of living with a violent abuser.

The Wheel is not a theory; it is a conceptual tool. It helps people see the patterns in behaviour and their significance. It is not intended to capture anything more than primary patterns, nor every tactic of control. The women did not identify a desire for power or control as motivating their partners to engage in these behaviours. Rather, abusers gained power and control in the relationship as an outcome of those behaviours. Underpinning many of these behaviours is an attitude of male rights, or entitlement.

The tactics do not in and of themselves constitute domestic violence. Abuse involves the patterned and intentional use of these tactics to control the victim's autonomy and deny her a life free of fear and intimidation. In short, asking a patient whether they are frightened of anyone may be the quickest way to begin a dialogue. Showing them the Wheel and asking whether anyone treats or has treated them in any of these ways can be very helpful.

In the UK, the Social Care Institute for Excellence (SCIE), through Department of Health funding, produced a free e-learning course for mental health professionals to help develop their confidence to ask service users questions and respond appropriately to promote their sexual and reproductive health, including their safety from abuse (see Resources on p. 48). It can be freely accessed by anyone as a learning tool to improve their practice. Module 3 on sexual and reproductive health is especially focused on good practice guidelines to address domestic violence.

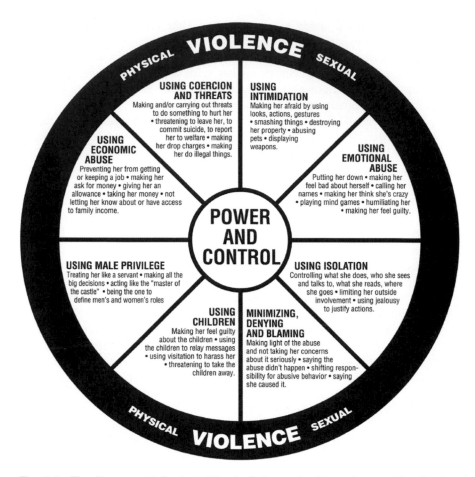

PHYSICAL **VIOLENCE** SEXUAL

USING COERCION AND THREATS
Making and/or carrying out threats to do something to hurt her • threatening to leave her, to commit suicide, to report her to welfare • making her drop charges • making her do illegal things.

USING INTIMIDATION
Making her afraid by using looks, actions, gestures • smashing things • destroying her property • abusing pets • displaying weapons.

USING ECONOMIC ABUSE
Preventing her from getting or keeping a job • making her ask for money • giving her an allowance • taking her money • not letting her know about or have access to family income.

USING EMOTIONAL ABUSE
Putting her down • making her feel bad about herself • calling her names • making her think she's crazy • playing mind games • humiliating her • making her feel guilty.

POWER AND CONTROL

USING MALE PRIVILEGE
Treating her like a servant • making all the big decisions • acting like the "master of the castle" • being the one to define men's and women's roles

USING ISOLATION
Controlling what she does, who she sees and talks to, what she reads, where she goes • limiting her outside involvement • using jealousy to justify actions.

USING CHILDREN
Making her feel guilty about the children • using the children to relay messages • using visitation to harass her • threatening to take the children away.

MINIMIZING, DENYING AND BLAMING
Making light of the abuse and not taking her concerns about it seriously • saying the abuse didn't happen • shifting responsibility for abusive behavior • saying she caused it.

PHYSICAL **VIOLENCE** SEXUAL

Fig. 3.2 The Power and Control Wheel. ©Domestic Abuse Intervention Project, reprinted with permission.

An alternative way to explore the pattern of the domestic violence is to ask about the first, the worst and the most recent incidents. You might ask whether the patient is scared of, or has been hurt by, more than one person or whether the abuse has happened more than once. Remember that some women face abuse from wider family and community networks so questions should not just focus on intimate partners. Thinking about any of these questions can help a patient to:

- understand the multiple aspects of abuse
- identify behaviours as domestic violence
- acknowledge the effects of violence on her mental health, and
- counteract her feeling of being alone or to blame.

It is important to remember that asking is not necessarily a one-off event. It may take a while for a woman who has experienced domestic violence to feel confident enough to respond to questions, if indeed she responds directly at all. She may use the information you provide without telling you.

Asking face to face *v.* self-completed measures

In the face of the evidence of under-detection of domestic violence by mental health professionals who rely on clinical interviews, self-completion questionnaires might increase disclosure rates. One large cluster randomised trial of different methods of screening for domestic violence in family practices, emergency departments and women's health clinics found that, when using the same standardised validated questionnaires, women preferred self-completed forms over face-to-face questioning (MacMillan *et al*, 2006). However, there is no evidence base on the use of self-completed measures in mental health services so it is not clear whether this is helpful or not. If self-completed measures are used the onus is on the clinician to continue the conversation and provide helpful support. One measure that has established validity and reliability and could therefore be considered for use in clinical settings is the Composite Abuse Scale, a 30-item self-report scale which includes the different types of abuse a woman may experience (Hegarty *et al*, 2005).

Improving cross-cultural understanding

Some service users are likely to encounter additional barriers when trying to access help because they have experienced discrimination or abuse elsewhere and/or are more vulnerable to entrapment as a function of their current situation. They will include victims who are Black, Asian or from another minority ethnic or refugee group; older or very young women; lesbian, gay or transgender; people with physical or intellectual disabilities; people who misuse drugs or alcohol; Gypsies or travellers; those working or forced to work in the sex industry; asylum seekers; or the homeless. In these cases, ask questions to establish a patient's isolation, the degree to which they are made vulnerable due to their dependency and their capacity to access social support (Box 3.7).

Box 3.7 Questions to consider when the patient is from a minority ethnic group

- Are you financially dependent?
- Have you any support networks or positive attachments outside the abusive relationship?
- Do you get to see/talk to family, friends or peers?
- Are you able to access agencies (general practitioner, health services, job centre, etc.)?
- Can you freely attend college/work/outside activities?
- Are you being pressurised to uphold family honour?
- Are you being told to do or not do things because of a cultural or religious responsibility?

When working with service users from a variety of communities it can help to phrase some of the questions using non-psychological terms (Rodriguez & Saba, 2006), as in these examples:

- What do you call your troubles?
- What do you fear most about your illness?
- When did your troubles begin?
- What or who makes things worse?
- What would be of most help to you?

The LEARN model to improve cross-cultural communication recommends:

1 *Listen* to the patient's perspective.
2 *Explain* and share your own view.
3 *Acknowledge* differences and similarities between the two views.
4 *Recommend* a specialist immigration support service.
5 *Never* accept culture as an excuse for domestic violence. Everyone deserves the right to be safe in their own home.

If the patient does not speak English as a first language, only professionally trained interpreters should be used for the assessment. It is important to remember that some women fear that any disclosure may reach their family through the interpreter owing to the tight-knit nature of some communities. Good practice guidance (Stella Project, 2009) recommends a cautious, common-sense approach when using an intepreter at patient assessment. This includes:

- never use a woman's partner, child, family member or 'friends';
- try to get a female interpreter where possible (if in an emergency this is not possible, do not press for details if you sense discomfort and try to arrange another time when a female interpreter is available);
- ask your interpreter to sign a confidentiality agreement;
- try not to use interpreters from a client's local area or from community associations to which she, her husband, family or friends may belong;
- contact an advocate from a specialist domestic violence agency;
- agree the agenda with the interpreter and that they will not 'edit' what the patient says;
- be alert to any discomfort or gaps in speech between the interpreter and patient (in either direction);
- look at your patient and speak directly to them, not the interpreter;
- have information available in an appropriate language.

Assessment in difficult situations

If the patient is always accompanied, it may demand resourcefulness or teamwork with a colleague to ensure that they have an opportunity to be interviewed alone. This might be particularly challenging if the index patient presents within a couple or family.

Perpetrators often use children to legitimise contact with ex-partners and as a vehicle to continue to harass or abuse them. In cases where parents have separated but domestic violence has been an issue, questions worth exploring with the patient may include (see also Resources, p. 48):

- Does he have parental responsibility?
- How many children, including any from a previous relationship, are there?
- Are there any formal or legal agreements about contact?
- Does he know where they go to school and after-school activities?
- Has he threatened to abduct or harm the children?
- Does he threaten that Social Services will remove the children?
- Does he threaten to send the children overseas?

It is also important to recognise and acknowledge that separation does not guarantee safety. Stalking or continued harassment have damaging effects on a victim's health. The following behaviours might be explored in an assessment. Has he:

- destroyed/vandalised property?
- turned up unannounced?
- loitered outside her work/college?
- called, emailed or texted obsessively?
- sent abusive letters?
- influenced others into berating or harassing her?
- entered the home when she was out?
- made threats? Of what kind?

Documentation

Writing down what the patient told you about domestic violence is an important aspect of treatment (Department of Health & Home Office, 2000; Williamson, 2000).

- It shows that you are listening and regard domestic violence as significant for mental health.
- Your records may be critical in criminal proceedings and can be required by statutory obligations (in the UK, under the Crime and Disorder Act 1998 (Section 115)).
- Your duty of care may be examined during a domestic homicide review, required by the Domestic Violence, Crime and Victims Act 2004.
- Your notes may play a crucial role in meeting a victim's legal rights, such as through an injunction to protect a vulnerable adult.
- You may help safeguard children at risk if an abuser attempts to continue harassment through contact or court orders.
- Your notes may be critical for addressing resettlement needs. Many housing agencies will accept a woman's application to be re-housed in a safe area if she can produce evidence that she has reported domestic violence to a mental health professional.

- You may help a victim access financial support or welfare rights.
- You will improve practice.

'What is important is that documentation is locally agreed and tested in order that there is ownership and commitment to its use. If documentation is onerous there will be disincentives for health professionals to identify cases of domestic violence. Paperwork should be the minimum necessary' (National Assembly for Wales, 2001: p. 30).

Records would ideally:
- always be made in an interview with the woman alone;
- include name, date of birth, ethnicity, number of children, pregnancy, friend or kin;
- include response to your questions about abuse;
- use the woman's own words when possible, rather than your own, using quotation marks or expressions such as 'patient reports' or 'Ms Smith said that' (not 'she claims' or 'alleges', which suggests you doubt it);
- briefly describe the types or nature of abuse;
- detail any physical impacts, including sketches of injury sites if possible;
- record, and if possible, keep, any damaged, torn or stained clothing;
- include dates and times of incidents, if known;
- include a description of patient's psychological state;
- document any relevant behaviour of the partner;
- describe detailed facts (including observations) rather than assumptions or summaries;
- record your action (e.g. safety planning, information provided, referral);
- be signed and dated, and have your name and role printed.

Sensitive information should not be included in letters or reports that may be seen by the perpetrator or a family member. The Department of Health (2010) recommends documenting 'violence not disclosed' where violence is denied.

Confidentiality

It is vital that information on domestic abuse is kept safe. Without confidentiality, women are less likely to talk about their experiences. Their physical safety can depend on it. All staff must understand and be honest about their efforts to maintain confidentiality, while being specific about their limitations (British Medical Association, 1998). Note that victims are primarily concerned about the abuser(s) rather than the clinical team finding out about the disclosure.

A woman's safety depends on notes being kept secure, including the patient's address, particularly if the abuser is registered with the same practice or hospital, or has potential access to National Health Service (NHS) data, including the NHS Spine.[1] Information sought over the telephone should always be preceded by a written and signed fax. Patients should be asked for permission to share information and have the value of sharing the information explained. (NB. Healthcare professionals should be aware that refuge[2] addresses are confidential and all residents are asked to maintain that confidentiality, although many women report being questioned and pressured by health professionals to reveal a street address.)

The clinician should explain to the patient that medical records are very important. They may help a victim to access legal rights, welfare rights, housing rights and thereby benefit them and the children in the longer term, even if not currently wanted by patients. The limits of confidentiality should also be explained at the beginning of a consultation – it is problematic to provide this information once a disclosure has been made.

Confidentiality could break down, for example, when using interpreters or dealing with requests for information from other professionals who may know the patient or come from the same community. Women from Black and minority ethnic and those from refugee communities may have concerns about sharing information with general practitioners who come from the same community as they fear confidentiality may be breached. Information should only be given to reputable agencies – never to individuals making enquiries about a woman's circumstances. If in doubt, ask for requests to be submitted in writing or by fax on headed paper.

When can information be shared without permission?

All actions around breaking patient confidentiality should be guided by the principle that the only acceptable reason for sharing information is to increase a woman's safety and/or that of her children. Even then, only share information that is relevant, on a need-to-know basis. Trust policy and multi-agency guidelines are available in relation to information-sharing and breaking patient confidentiality with and without consent. If information is passed on without permission, this should not place somebody at risk of greater violence. It can be helpful to encourage the patient to share the information herself and offer to support her, for instance by explaining that often the best way to support children at risk of domestic violence is

---

1   The NHS Spine is a national information service that stores patient information including their name, address, date of birth and summarised clinical information. While intended to help access to information to improve healthcare, it may be vulnerable to misuse by abusers intent on locating a victim.

2   Refuges are safe houses or temporary accommodation for victims of domestic violence. They use a mailbox and postcode rather than a street address to reduce the risk of residents being tracked down and further abused. Health professionals need to be aware that a resident is complying with house safety rules, not being evasive, if they offer a mailbox number.

to promote the safety of the non-abusive parent, or that it is the violence rather than the patient that is the problem. However, if the patient does not agree to information-sharing, a supervisor or manager should be consulted as it is not always easy to balance confidentiality against the interests of disclosure. A patient should be told whenever information has been shared.

According to current UK legislation (Section 115 of the Crime and Disorder Act 1998), it is permissible to pass information to another agency without consent in situations where:

(a) the court requests information about a specific case; or
(b) there is significant risk of harm to the woman, her children or somebody else if information is not passed on (Department of Health, 2005, p. 81).

For more information, see guidance in the Home Office's document *Safety and Justice: Sharing Personal Information in the Context of Domestic Violence* (Douglas *et al*, 2004).

Never help a partner locate a victim if she has left him. Do not pass on letters, messages or facilitate contact with an alleged perpetrator of domestic violence – clinicians and service users could be put in danger. If children are at risk, local safeguarding or child protection policies should be followed (see also Chapter 6).

Conclusions

Mental health service users are at increased risk of domestic violence but their experiences are often undetected by mental health professionals. Professionals should be trained how to routinely enquire about domestic violence and know how to respond safely to disclosures.

This chapter has discussed how to identify domestic violence and the following chapter will discuss appropriate responses to disclosures.

References

Bacchus, L., Mezey, G. & Bewley, S. (2008) Women's perceptions and experiences of routine enquiry for domestic violence in a maternity service. *International Journal of Obstetrics and Gynaecology*, **109**, 9–16.

Barnish, M. (2004) *Domestic Violence: A Literature Review*. HM Inspectorate of Probation.

Bewley, S., Friend, J. & Mezey, G. (1997) *Violence Against Women*. Royal College of Obstetricians and Gynaecologists.

British Medical Association (1998) *Domestic Violence: A Health Care Issue?* British Medical Association.

British Medical Association (2007) *Domestic Abuse: A Report from the British Medical Association Board of Science*. British Medical Association.

Department of Health (2005) *Responding to Domestic Abuse: A Handbook for Health Professionals*. TSO (The Stationery Office).

Department of Health (2008) *Refocusing the Care Programme Approach: Policy and Positive Practice Guidance*. Department of Health.

Department of Health (2009) *Improving Safety, Reducing Harm: Children, Young People and Domestic Violence – A Practical Toolkit for Front-line Practitioners*. TSO (The Stationery Office).

Department of Health (2010) *Responding to Violence Against Women and Children – The Role of the NHS*. Department of Health.

Department of Health & Home Office (2000) *No Secrets: Guidance on Developing and Implementing Multi-Agency Policies and Procedures to Protect Vulnerable Adults from Abuse.* Department of Health.

Douglas, N., Lilley, S.-J., Kooper, L., *et al* (2004) *Safety and Justice: Sharing Personal Information in the Context of Domestic Violence – An Overview*. Home Office Research, Development and Statistics Directorate.

Ethnic Alcohol Counselling in Hounslow (EACH) (2009) *Asian Women, Domestic Violence and Mental Health: A Toolkit for Health Professionals*. EACH.

Feder, G., Hutson, M., Ramsay, J., *et al* (2006) Women exposed to intimate partner violence: expectations and experiences when they encounter health-care professionals: a meta-analysis of qualitative studies. *Annals of Internal Medicine*, **166**, 22–37.

Feder, G., Ramsay, J., Dunne, D., *et al* (2009) How far does screening women for domestic (partner) violence in different health-care settings meet criteria for a screening programme? Systematic reviews of nine UK, National Screening Committee critieria. *Health Technology Assessment*, **13**, iii–113.

Foreign & Commonwealth Office (2007) *Dealing with Cases of Forced Marriage: Practice Guidance for Health Professionals* (1st edn). FCO Services: publishing.

Gill, A. (2004) Voicing the silent fear: south asian women's experiences of domestic violence. *The Howard Journal of Criminal Justice*, **43**, 465–483.

Goodman, L. A., Thompson, K. M., Weinfurt, K., *et al* (1999) Reliability of reports of violent victimization and posttraumatic stress disorder among men and women with serious mental illness. *Journal of Traumatic Stress*, **12**, 587–599.

Greater London Domestic Violence Project (2008) *Sane Responses: Good Practice Guidelines for Domestic Violence and Mental Health Services*. Greater London Domestic Violence Project.

Harris, V., Loise, R., Spencer, H., *et al* (2002) *Domestic Abuse Screening Pilot in Primary Care 2000–2002 Final Report*. Support & Survival.

Hegarty, K., Bush, R. & Sheehan, M. (2005) The Composite Abuse Scale: further development and assessment of reliability and validity of a multidimensional partner abuse measure in clinical settings. *Violence and Victims*, **20**, 529–547.

Howard, L. M., Trevillion, K., Khalifeh, H., *et al* (2010) Domestic violence and severe psychiatric disorders: prevalence and interventions. *Psychological Medicine*, **40**, 881–893.

MacMillan, L. H., Wathen, C. N., Jamieson, E., *et al* (2006) Approaches to screening for intimate partner violence in health care settings: a randomized trial. *JAMA*, **296**, 530–536.

Mullender, A., Hague, G., Imam, U., *et al* (2002) *Children's Perspectives on Domestic Violence*. Sage Publications.

National Assembly for Wales (2001) *Domestic Violence: A Resource Manual for Health Care Professionals in Wales*. National Assembly for Wales.

Oram, S., Trevillion, K., Feder, G., *et al* (2013) Prevalence of experiences of domestic violence among psychiatric patients: systematic review. *British Journal of Psychiatry*, **202**, 94–99.

Pence, E. & Paymar, M. (1986) *Power and Control: Tactics of Men who Batter*. Minnesota Program Development.

Rai, D. K. & Thiara, R. K. (1997) *Redefining Spaces: The Needs of Black Women and Children in Refuge Support Services and Black Workers in Women's Aid*. Women's Aid Federation of England.

Ramsay, J., Richardson, J., Carter, Y. H., *et al* (2002) Should health professionals screen for domestic violence? Systematic review. *BMJ*, **325**, 1–13.

Read, J., van Os, J., Morrison, A., *et al* (2005) Childhood trauma, psychosis and schizophrenia: a literature review with theoretical and clinical implications. *Acta Psychiatrica Scandinavica*, **112**, 330–350.

Rodriguez, M. A. & Saba, G. (2006) Cultural competence and intimate partner abuse: health care interventions. In *Intimate Partner Abuse and Health Professionals. New Approaches to Domestic Violence* (eds G. Roberts, K. Hegarty & G. Feder), pp. 181–196. Churchill Livingstone Elsevier.

Rose, D., Trevillion, K., Woodall, A., *et al* (2011) Barriers and facilitators of disclosures of domestic violence by mental health service users: qualitative study. *British Journal of Psychiatry*, **198**, 189–194.

Social Care Institute for Excellence (2011) eLearning: Sexual, reproductive and mental health. SCIE (http://www.scie.org.uk/publications/elearning/sexualhealth/index.asp).

Stella Project (2009) *Domestic Violence, Drugs and Alcohol: Good Practice Guidelines* (2nd edn). Against Violence and Abuse (AVA).

Taket, A., Nurse, J., Smith, K., *et al* (2003) Routinely asking women about domestic violence in health settings. *BMJ*, **327**, 673–676.

Taskforce on the Health Aspects of Violence against Women and Children (2010) *Report from the Domestic Violence sub-group: Responding to Violence against Women and Children – The Role of the NHS*. Department of Health.

Trevillion, K., Agnew-Davies, R. & Howard, L. M. (2010) Domestic violence: responding to the needs of patients. *Nursing Standard*, **25**, 48–56.

Trevillion, K., Howard, L. M., Morgan, C., *et al* (2012) The response of mental health services to domestic violence: a qualitative study of service users' and professionals' experiences. *Journal of the American Psychiatric Nurses Association*, epub ahead of print, doi: 10.1177/1078390312459747.

Williamson, E. (2000) *Domestic Violence and Health: The Response of the Medical Profession*. Policy Press.

Zweig, J. M., Schlichter, K. A. & Burt, M. R. (2002) Assisting women victims of violence who experience multiple barriers to services. *Violence Against Women*, **8**, 162–180.

Resources

If you have concerns about identifying or discussing experiences with a patient whom you think might be at risk, there are a number of toolkits and practice guidance you can download or agencies that could help guide you what to ask (see also Appendix 2).

The Duluth wheel for using children post-separation: www.theduluthmodel.org/cms/files/UsingChildrenPostSeparation.pdf

Forced marriage practice guidance issued by UK government: www.gov.uk/government/uploads/system/uploads/attachment_data/file/35530/forced-marriage-guidelines09.pdf

Sane Responses: a mental health and domestic violence toolkit from AVA (Against Violence & Abuse): www.avaproject.org.uk/our-resources/good-practice-guidance--toolkits/sane-responses-good-practice-guidelines-for-domestic-violence-and-mental-health-services-(2008).aspx

SCIE programme for mental health professionals on managing patients' reproductive health: www.scie.org.uk/assets/elearning/sexualhealth/Web/Object3/main.html

Stella Project Toolkit: drugs, alcohol and domestic violence toolkit from AVA for health and domestic violence workers: www.avaproject.org.uk/our-resources/good-practice-guidance--toolkits/stella-project-toolkit-(2007).aspx

Toolkit for working with children and young people from the Department of Health: www.dh.gov.uk/en/Publicationsandstatistics/Publications/PublicationsPolicyAndGuidance/DH_108697

CHAPTER 4

Responding to disclosures of domestic violence

Roxane Agnew-Davies

Many clinicians either respond inappropriately or feel ill equipped or lacking in training to respond to disclosures about domestic violence from service users. Because the healthcare system may be the victim's first or only point of contact with professionals (Donaldson & Marshall, 2005), the initial response of a mental health professional after any disclosure is crucial to promote the person's safety, access to appropriate support and recovery. As in Chapter 3, most of this chapter is based on good practice guidelines for female victims of domestic violence, as there is a very limited evidence base on the optimal response of mental health professionals and most literature refers to women, reflecting the higher prevalence and severity of violence and abuse experienced by women. This work also draws from feedback from service users on what they found helpful or unhelpful about mental health professionals' responses to initial disclosures of experiences of abuse (Feder *et al*, 2006; Rose *et al*, 2011; Trevillion *et al*, 2012). As in Chapter 3, the good practice guidance refers to clinicians working with colleagues in the multidisciplinary team. Healthcare professionals should not attempt to manage a disclosure of domestic violence alone; discussion of the complex issues involved is helpful, and multidisciplinary support in the assessment, formulation and management of patients is essential.

What service users want to hear

Women who have experienced domestic violence have been asked to identify what would be a positive initial response to disclosure (Rodriguez *et al*, 1996). They came up with several issues: creating a supportive environment, providing continued support, developing trust and reassurance of confidentiality. From other studies, it emerged that what is also important is information-giving, making referrals to community resources or providing resources on site; talking about the violence in a compassionate and sensitive manner; promoting safety; documenting the abuse; and a non-judgemental response (McNutt *et al*, 1999; Rose *et al*, 2011). Women have emphasised the need for health professionals to listen to their concerns, respond in a non-judgemental and non-directive way and work at a pace at which they felt comfortable, without pressing for a quick resolution of the problem (Feder *et al*, 2006). Body language and facial expressions were subtle but important ways of showing concern and developing trust (Rodriguez *et al*, 1996). The most frequently reported concern was that the health professional would medicalise the issues or take control of the situation without the woman's permission, for example, by calling the police or by discussing the abuse with the perpetrator present (McNutt *et al*, 1999; Feder *et al*, 2006). A first principle in health practice is to do no harm. In relation to domestic violence, harmful responses include ignoring the abuse, blaming the victim, medicalising psychological reactions without relating them to the abuse experienced and letting the perpetrator know about the disclosure so that the patient is at risk of further harm. This is further outlined in Table 4.1.

Table 4.1 Helpful and unhelpful responses to domestic violence disclosures

Helpful	Unhelpful	Your role
Help to name domestic violence and hold perpetrator accountable	Failing to recognise the abuse; blaming the victim; focusing on the relationship not the abuse	Be aware of the signs, ask questions about abuse (see Chapter 3); identify the abuse as the problem; make it easier to talk about experiences
Give attention to risk and focus on safety of victim and children	Reacting with disbelief or scepticism, telling her what to do; suggesting family therapy or couple counselling involving the perpetrator	Be knowledgeable about key risks; record evidence; do not talk to a victim about abuse in presence of an abuser; explore how a victim can put in place a plan to increase safety
Respond to special needs	Focusing simply on medication or substance use without recognising the complexity of partner violence; working in isolation	Be prepared to work in partnership with other agencies; have information available in different formats; acknowledge the complexities and long-term nature of abuse
Help recovery from experiences of abuse	Making the abuser invisible by focusing only on the victim's mental health	Be non-judgemental; set the symptoms in the context of trauma; hold the abuser not the victim accountable; acknowledge her range of survival strategies
Offer support for children	Focusing on failure to protect children rather than the source of abuse	Give information and refer her to relevant agencies with her consent; promote children's well-being by support for the non-abusive parent
Recognise stages of change	Withholding treatment because the victim is living in an abusive situation	Adapt intervention to suit needs and stage; risk assess and safety plan, or refer to someone who can

What should you say next? Key messages after disclosure

Since a health professional may be the only person to whom a woman discloses her experience of domestic violence, it is critical that the first response includes some key messages. Examples are given below and further examples can be explored in a free e-learning resource for mental health professionals available on the UK Social Care Institute for Excellence website about sexual and reproductive health, including good practice in addressing abuse (see Resources in Chapter 3, p. 48, for more information).

1. The disclosure is helpful and important

Health professionals with expertise in domestic violence validate a woman's experience and express solidarity before any other response (Feder *et al*, 2005). Let her feel that you are pleased to know, for instance, by thanking her for trusting you, or by saying that you think it was important that she told you because domestic violence can be very damaging to her health. You might mention that it took courage, or that you appreciate her openness, especially as someone in her life has previously abused that trust. You could acknowledge that while there may be a lot to talk through, it cannot all be resolved at once (by either of you). Offer ongoing support and indicate that you are willing to talk to her again. Explore safe ways to remain in contact: where she can be reached, whether it is safe for you to call or write to her at home, whether you need to agree a code when you call (e.g. you could say it is the GP's receptionist if the abuser answers the phone) or perhaps she has a safe contact number in case of emergency.

2. She is not alone and it is not her fault

Often victims feel isolation, shame and self-blame which may have been engendered by their partner or family members. It can be useful to point out that her feelings, behaviour and problems are the result rather than the cause of domestic violence. Through enhancing your understanding of the prevalence and nature of abuse, you can reassure the service user that domestic violence is widespread; this knowledge alone can help counteract her feelings. See Chapter 1 for some useful statistics you could share with her (e.g. pp. 5–8).

The abuser, not the victim, is responsible for the violence; nothing anyone has said or done justifies physical or sexual abuse. It is critical that a professional does not ask questions about how she may have provoked the abuser that could account for the violence. The victim of violence is not the cause of the violence (Hegarty, 2005).

Key messages should highlight that domestic violence is unacceptable; that perpetrators alone are responsible for the abuse; and that substance use, stress, the abuser's childhood or external factors do not explain or excuse violence. While there is a correlation between these factors and perpetration or victimisation of abuse, the majority of people with these problems are not violent to their partners or families (Barnish, 2004).

3. Service users with mental health problems have the right to be safe. Domestic violence can negatively affect mental health

A failure to identify the aetiology of mental health symptoms can be compounded by an abusive partner or family member who attributes problems to the victim's mental health or behaviour. These issues have potential for further victimisation (Feder *et al*, 2005), including inappropriate management of service users who are experiencing abuse. There are at least two key messages that any mental health professional might convey. First, domestic violence causes not only physical injury but psychological trauma and second, that people with mental health problems have the same right to be safe as anyone else.

4. Safety at home is a priority

Freedom from assault is every person's basic right. Domestic violence can cause serious injury or death. Women at or just after the point of separation are at most risk from an escalation of physical violence or threats to their life (Richards, 2006). Professionals can assure a service user of the right to be safe in their home and offer to explore means to improve their protection. This might not mean leaving the family home. Risk assessment and safety planning is discussed later on (pp. 56–62).

Trauma-focused therapy will only be effective when the service user feels safe and secure in their living environment, to a degree sufficient to withstand the emotional intensity of re-exposure to trauma and cognitive re-processing. Research into successful treatment of service users suffering from post-traumatic stress disorder (PTSD) has demonstrated the necessity of a three-staged model of care (e.g. Herman, 1998; Zimmerman *et al*, 2006), particularly for victims of prolonged abuse. The three stages are:

1   crisis/emergency intervention;
2   support, recuperation and psychological adjustment; and
3   long-term symptom management.

This is not to say that the mental health professional should refuse treatment until the service user is safe; on the contrary, this would effectively collude with the abuser and leave them isolated and at risk. The role of the mental health professional is to offer information and support to access domestic violence services if a service user is at risk.

5. There is help available

A number of agencies can help a person take steps to ensure their safety, irrespective of a decision to stay in or leave the relationship. Offer a telephone in a private space and have ready a list of national helpline numbers as well as local services and referral pathways. The free 24-hour National Domestic Violence Helpline (run in partnership by Refuge and Women's Aid) is 0808 2000 247. Trained staff and volunteers can listen to the person and offer them confidential emotional support; give information on housing, welfare, health and legal rights; refer women and children to refuges (places of safety) or make referrals to temporary emergency accommodation; and advocate on behalf of women to access support from police, emergency services, support agencies and specialist services. Service users may prefer to visit www.womensaid.org.uk or www.refuge.org.uk to find out more. For male victims there is also the men's advice line: 0808 801 0327, website: www.mensadviceline.org.uk; and for lesbian, gay, bisexual or transgender people there is a specialist telephone line operated by Broken Rainbow: 0300 999 5428, website: www.broken-rainbow.org.uk. All these organisations can put people in touch with local services (see Appendix 2 for a list of such organisations with contact details).

6. Service users have the right to talk about abuse in privacy

Talking about domestic violence can feel difficult (see Chapter 3). Discuss the options and use principles that match appropriate responses to disclosure of abuse. Assure service users of confidentiality when possible (in that you will not discuss their disclosures with the perpetrator/perpetrators or family members) and the benefits of any disclosure, such as improving future access to legal, welfare and housing rights.

7. The service user is the expert by experience

The clinician's role is to empower service users to make their own choices, but the service user must lead the process of change. She is the only person who can know what is best for her and the only person who has all the information about her situation.

- **Do not try to make decisions for her.** It is crucial that she decides herself what it is she wants to do next. Do not, for instance, tell her that she must leave her partner. She may not feel ready, safe or may not want to do this. Telling her what to do might compound her isolation and fears about approaching 'outsiders' for help in the future. It also might jeopardise her safety.
- **Ask her what she wants you to do.** Be clear about what is possible, but explain that other agencies might be able to help in areas where you cannot.
- **Discuss options.** These might include seeking advice from a helpline; getting support from domestic violence agencies; staying in hospital overnight; contacting the police; getting legal advice about obtaining an injunction or restraining order; seeking emergency refuge accommodation; making a safety plan.
- **Support the patient in whatever decision they make.** You might not understand her decision. She might decide to stay with or return to

an abuser – and not just because she is afraid to leave him. Sometimes women still love their abuser, believe he can change or want their children to grow up with their father.

- **Do not judge her or make assumptions.** For example, if she is from a minority ethnic background, do not assume that she will only accept help from culturally specific agencies. Do not assume that a victim would necessarily prefer to talk to a woman; although you might offer that choice if possible, many victims have felt empowered by a male professional stating that abuse is unacceptable.

8. Service users may be already trying to change the situation and promote their safety

One of the most positive responses you can make is to recognise a service user's own efforts to change the situation. Very few victims give up trying to change their situation, in all sorts of ways. They adopt survival techniques, make active decisions and develop conscious or unconscious ways of coping, which are often missed or unacknowledged by health professionals (Table 4.2).

Table 4.2 Common survival strategies

Type of strategy	Examples of actions a victim takes
Legal strategies	Calls police; contacts solicitor; seeks injunctions
Formal help-seeking	Approaches statutory agencies (healthcare, Social Services, housing) or voluntary organisations (refuge, helpline, advice centre)
Informal help-seeking	Talks to friends, family; asks neighbour to call police; asks relative to intervene, directly (to speak to abuser) or indirectly (to be present)
Escape behaviours	Walks away, barricades a room; flees house; goes to public place with CCTV; runs to mother's house
Separation	Moves out; applies for divorce
Hiding	Tries to keep address of home, work or school secret; disguises appearance; changes name
Appeals to abuser	Talks to 'calm him down'; asks him to promise to stop; asks him to explain; tries to distract or divert
Compliance	Anticipates abuser's demands: does things to please or avoids doing things she believes might trigger violence; complies with demands (e.g. has sex 'to keep the peace')
Resistance	Answers back; threatens action (e.g. to call police); attempts suicide
Self-defence	Passive (blocking, resisting) and active (striking)
Manages children	Asks children to call police, to seek help, to leave; asks children to comply to protect against abuse
Personal	Dissociates; relies on religious convictions

There is no single effective strategy for all victims. Some strategies that seem useful in theory (e.g. calling police) may not work in practice; many women say their partner will not be deterred or that police cannot keep a 24-hour watch. Some strategies may result in an increase in violence or negative consequences (e.g. a woman is ostracised for leaving a violent husband) and a strategy that works once might not work when tried again. No strategy is used in isolation and victims typically use a combination, which vary across time.

9. A good father does not put his children at risk

There is clear evidence that children suffer emotional and psychological impacts of witnessing abuse, as well as the possibility they may also be at risk of physical harm (see Chapter 1, pp. 12–13). Child protection guidance recognises that witnessing domestic abuse can cause significant harm and children in families in which domestic violence is occurring must be regarded as children in need of safeguarding. In relationships where there is domestic violence, children witness about three-quarters of the abusive incidents. About half the children in such families have themselves been badly hit or beaten and are more likely to be victims of sexual and emotional abuse (see Chapter 1).

However, to avoid a 'victim-blaming' approach when addressing risks to children with patients, professionals are advised to tackle the topic with sensitivity, respect and clarity that it is the perpetrator, not the non-abusive parent, who is the cause of the abuse. Many victims have been threatened that their children will be removed and inadvertently blamed for failing to protect their child, whereas the abuser is neither challenged nor charged. It is critical for your patient who is at risk to understand that your primary concern is to safeguard them and the children.

10. Domestic violence is against the law

Domestic violence undermines an individual's human rights and the behaviours that constitute domestic violence, such as harassment, threats to kill and assaults are recognised crimes. However, many women are unaware of their legal rights or do not know that the behaviours which characterise domestic violence are criminal. Others understand that their abuser does not respect the law, but they may not be aware that breaching court orders can now incur up to 5 years' imprisonment in the UK.

Collaboration with other members of the team and other agencies

Effective responses to domestic violence are not simply a conversation with a patient but depend on effective multidisciplinary teamwork and multi-agency collaboration. This also prevents the health professional from straying beyond their level of competence and shields them from feeling solely responsible for the safety of the victim. No one can work with domestic violence alone.

A unique and probably essential feature of the successful Identification and Referral to Improve Safety (IRIS) model trialled in UK primary care settings (Feder *et al*, 2011) was close partnership with third-sector specialist agencies. The IRIS model promoted inter-agency communication between primary care practitioners and a named advocate educator based in a local domestic violence service. The advocate educator trained practices in the identification of, and response to, women who experience domestic violence, and became the named advocate to whom clinicians could refer. Domestic violence advocates are trained to conduct risk assessments and to help victims of domestic violence with safety planning, although clinicians can support these processes. A pilot study of a partnership with reciprocal training and a direct referral pathway involving community mental health teams and domestic violence advocates in south-east London (the LARA study) has reported improved outcomes for service users (decreased unmet needs and experiences of abuse, and improved quality of life), improvements in knowledge of practitioners and increased rates of referrals to Multi-Agency Risk Assessment Conferences (MARACs) (data available from the author on request). There is therefore preliminary evidence that partnership with domestic violence services (such as referral pathways from primary care to domestic violence advocates in local services) can improve mental health outcomes for service users and increase competencies of staff.

Risk assessment and safety planning to prevent or reduce domestic violence

'The key to responding effectively to domestic abuse is to understand risk assessment and safety planning as interlinked processes' (Department of Health, 2009: p. 121).

Many women who experience domestic violence are aware of the danger they are in and have already developed a range of strategies to aid their protection (see Table 4.2, p. 54). They may also have thought about and begun to make plans for escape in a crisis. For others, the opportunity you create to discuss the risk of further harm (risk assessment) may reveal a pattern (such as escalation in the frequency or severity of abuse) of which she had not been aware and indicate that you care about her safety. Risk assessment is an integral part of all mental health assessments, of course, but to date there has been limited focus on the specific risks associated with abuse (Trevillion *et al*, 2012). The discussion about what she then needs to do (safety planning) must be integral to this recognition. A domestic violence advisor can assist in both risk assessment and safety planning. Although many perpetrators of domestic violence are only violent to their partners, relatives and children, the possibility that he may present a risk to the clinician should also be considered, especially if mental health contacts take place in the family home.

The Department of Health (2005) guidance *Responding to Domestic Abuse* identifies three stages of risk assessment that are relevant to health professionals:

1   an immediate risk assessment between the professional and the service user when domestic violence has been disclosed;
2   an organisational assessment linked to wider trust and safeguarding policies; and
3   broader multi-agency risk assessment, for example through MARACs.

There is also a fourth form of specialised risk assessment when a specialist domestic violence advocate or expert mental health professional prepares a detailed or forensic risk assessment report. A local independent domestic violence advocate (IDVA) can help a service user assess risk and draw up a safety plan. Contact the National Domestic Violence Helpline (tel. 0808 2000 247) or even better, find out and keep ready the numbers for your local domestic violence coordinator or agency.

Initial assessment

A preliminary risk assessment, when the service user needs an emergency decision about whether they or the children may be at risk of immediate harm, could include these questions:

*   Is it safe for you to go home?
*   What are you afraid might happen?
*   What has the abuser threatened?
*   What about threats to the children?

Any mental health professional can encourage women to contact a specialist domestic violence service for more comprehensive assessments of risk, detailed safety planning and ongoing support. Any decisions to leave the home or relationship must be raised in the knowledge that most domestic violence homicides of women occur at or around the point of separation. Careful discussion and planning, with specialist support, is important at this stage.

Further risk assessment

A number of tools are currently used to assess risk to women and children. These tools explore many risk factors and may help mental health professionals when carrying out assessments. They are not a replacement for clinical assessment, which should not be a standalone tick-box task, but the beginning of a dialogue with the victim, in conjunction with other information. Risk is not static and low risk can change rapidly, so assessments must be dynamic and constantly reviewed and updated.

British Crime Surveys (e.g. Walby & Myhill, 2000) and the Metropolitan Police Service murder reviews (Richards, 2006; Richards *et al*, 2008; Stobart, 2009) have identified key areas of potential danger, later collated into the DASH checklist. The acronym DASH stands for Domestic Abuse, Stalking and Honour Based Violence, and the checklist was originally developed by Laura Richards, a forensic psychologist (Richards *et al*, 2008). It was shortened by Co-ordinated Action Against Domestic Abuse (CAADA) into a risk assessment checklist used by domestic violence advocates and MARACs (see Appendix 1). The DASH checklist has been subjected to rigorous examination and cross-validation. The more issues that apply, the higher the risk of severe injury or homicide. Note that risk factors are not causal factors. Mental health problems, experienced by either the victim or the perpetrator, are included in this list. In addition, you might ask about:

- disputes over child contact;
- sexual abuse;
- previous assault/abuse;
- escalation in severity or frequency of violence;
- ongoing harassment or stalking;
- recent or planned separation;
- threats/attempts to kill/die by suicide (by either partner);
- pregnancy or young children;
- previous criminal behaviour;
- child abuse;
- substance misuse;
- morbid jealousy (e.g. unjust accusations of infidelity, 'policing', instructing what clothes to wear);
- any abuse or harassment by people other than the primary perpetrator;
- victim vulnerabilities, such as isolation.

After assessing immediate safety, risk assessment should address the history of abuse (physical, emotional or sexual) including the impact(s) on children. In particular, has the violence increased in intensity, frequency and/or severity? One way to evaluate escalation may be to ask about first, worst and last episodes of abuse. More specific questions are:

- Does he threaten to kill her and/or does she believe he is capable of killing her?
- What has he threatened to do?
- Has he ever threatened her with a weapon or used a weapon?
- Does he ever try to choke her or put his hands around her throat?
- Has he ever forced sex, or made her do sexual things that she did not want to do?
- Has she been beaten while pregnant, now or in the past?
- Has he ever harmed the children? Does he threaten to harm them or take them?
- Is he violent outside the home, for example, has he frightened or threatened friends or family?

- Does he control most or all of her daily activities? For instance, to whom she can talk, how much money she can have or when she can use the phone?
- Is he possessive or jealous? For example, has he said, 'If I can't have you, no one can!'?
- Has he ever threatened or tried to die by suicide?
- In what ways is mental or emotional abuse putting her at risk, for example of suicide or self-harm?

A risk assessment can also explore factors that might mitigate against abuse and inform a safety plan. For example:

- Has she had help (e.g. from police, courts, domestic violence services) and what was the response? Does she know about legal, welfare or housing rights?
- Who could offer emotional or practical support (e.g. friends, family, neighbours)?
- Does she have access to money or benefits in an emergency?
- Is safe alternative accommodation available if she does not want to return home?

The person who is experiencing the violence is ultimately the only one who can reliably predict the risks they are facing. The clinician's principal role is to support them in the decisions and choices they wish to make.

Safeguarding children

Under the UK Adoption and Children Act 2002, living with and witnessing domestic violence is identified as a source of 'significant harm' for children. As will be discussed in Chapter 6 (pp. 82–84), trust or local authority safeguarding children guidelines must be followed if there are children in the family. Risk assessments should focus on the emotional and developmental needs of the child as well as their health and physical safety. Questions should be asked about the children's whereabouts when the abuse occurs, whether they intervene, whether they are ever directly threatened or hurt and the impact on their routines, health, relationships and education. If children are at risk, child protection guidelines must be followed. Supporting the non-abusive parent to be safe and supporting her parenting can be the most effective form of child protection. The need to follow these procedures can be discussed with the patient and their consent obtained, if possible. However, the interests of the child are paramount, and initiating procedures is not conditional on obtaining consent.

More information about children and domestic violence, including risk assessment questions and templates for safety planning with children and young people, can be found in a toolkit prepared by the Department of Health (2009), *Improving Safety, Reducing Harm: Children, Young People and Domestic Violence: A Practical Toolkit for Front-Line Practitioners*.

Risk assessment and diversity

There are many barriers to women accessing support (individual, practical, social and cultural) that can compound reactions to the violence (Dutton, 1992) and compromise safety.

- Patients with intellectual or physical disabilities may be dependent on a caregiver, and psychological abuse may have further undermined their capacity for independence. Service users with these issues may feel obliged to be grateful and more vulnerable to shame or blame.
- Additional life stressors, for example risk of social exclusion, language barriers, insecure immigration status with the threat of deportation (and/or ostracism or harm if they were returned). A woman's community may not accept divorce or separation. Young Asian women may be at particular risk of significant harm following disclosure, and special care should be given to their safety (Stobart, 2009).
- Risk factors associated with dowry abuse, forced marriage and dowry-related violence, including the risk of 'honour killing'.
- A woman may be afraid of being rejected by her family or the wider community if she leaves. For example, lesbian women may fear discrimination, loss of support or loss of their children if their sexuality is 'outed'.

These issues should be given attention when assessing risk and safety planning.

Safety planning

Increasing safety and escaping domestic violence may be a slow and incremental process (James-Hanman, 1998). Women may leave and return a number of times. Even while they remain in an abusive situation, they can still be making important changes and it does not mean that your help has been wasted or that your patient is not taking action. It is extremely important that you do not withhold treatment just because the patient is unwilling to end a violent relationship; as has emerged from research on stages of change, the clinician needs to tailor the intervention to meet the patient's current needs. While they are at risk, this will include information, partnership work and referral for advocacy. Even if your patient returns to a violent partner, she may view the situation differently, she may act differently if the violence re-occurs and she may have prepared to take action or make changes in her life to free herself from violence. Moreover, the relationship is not the same as the abuse – she is returning to the former, not the latter.

Whether or not she chooses to leave her partner, her safety is the most important thing. The role of the professional is not to cajole, advise or insist; it is more important that the choice is always the patient's, and that the door remains open for her to talk some more when she is ready. The

Department of Health guidelines (Department of Health, 2005) suggest that a safety plan should cover the following points:

1   Safety in the relationship:
    - places to avoid when abuse starts (such as the kitchen, with potential weapons);
    - people a woman can turn to for help or let know that she is in danger;
    - asking neighbours or friends to call 999 if they hear anything to suggest a woman or her children are in danger;
    - places to hide important phone numbers, such as helpline numbers;
    - how to keep the children safe when abuse starts;
    - teaching the children to find safety or get help, perhaps by dialling 999;
    - keeping important personal documents in one place so that they can be taken if a woman needs to leave suddenly;
    - letting someone know about the abuse so that it can be recorded (important for cases that go to court or immigration applications, for example).

2   Leaving in an emergency:
    - packing an emergency bag and hiding it in a safe place in case a woman needs to leave in an emergency;
    - plans for who to call and where to go (such as a domestic violence refuge);
    - things to remember to take: documents, medication, keys or a photo of the abuser (useful for serving court documents);
    - access to a telephone;
    - access to money or credit/debit cards that a woman has perhaps put aside;
    - plans for transport;
    - plans for taking clothes, toiletries and toys for the children;
    - taking any proof of the abuse, such as photos, notes or details of people who know about it.

3   Safety when a relationship is over:
    - contact details for professionals who can advise or give vital support;
    - changing landline and mobile telephone numbers;
    - how to keep her location secret from her partner if she has left home (e.g. by not telling mutual friends where she is);
    - obtaining a non-molestation, exclusion or restraining order;
    - plans for talking to children about the importance of staying safe;
    - asking her employer for help with safety while at work.

It is also important to help her to focus on the more positive things going on in her life and/or identify ways in which she could access activities which would help improve her confidence, self-esteem and emotional well-being.

Longer-term strategies

Professionals can help a woman affected by domestic violence restore her longer-term safety and empowerment by:

- encouraging her to recognise or regain her personal strengths and competencies;
- addressing specific needs, for example substance misuse;
- increasing her access to resources, through information (e.g. about welfare benefits) or discussing safe options for places to stay;
- facilitating her aim for financial independence, through seeking employment or retraining; plans for saving prior to the escape;
- discussing her legal rights and explaining her rights to her property;
- increasing her social support to develop affiliation, perspective and comfort outside the abusive relationship; encouraging the woman to widen her network by beginning or renewing contact with friends, family, cultural groups, hospital groups, classes;
- offering wider professional support to increasing her range of options and sources of support, for example, a domestic violence helpline, local voluntary sector agencies, Social Services, housing services, a solicitor and the Department for Work and Pensions, or similar agencies;
- helping her with safe management of contact arrangements to minimise risk and distress.

Conclusions

Key messages confirm the right for everyone to feel safe and attribute responsibility for the abuse to the perpetrator rather than the victim. Good practice requires the practitioner to ask patients whether they would like to be referred to domestic violence specialists, and to check immediate risk to the service user and children. If some degree of risk is detected, mental health professionals can help service users explore or rehearse safety planning in the context of understanding stages of change and previously used strategies to promote their own protection.

References

Barnish, M. (2004) *Domestic Violence: A Literature Review*. HM Inspectorate of Probation.

Department of Health (2005) *Responding to Domestic Abuse: A Handbook for Health Professionals*. Department of Health.

Department of Health (2009) *Improving Safety, Reducing Harm: Children, Young People and Domestic Violence: A Practical Toolkit for Front-Line Practitioners*. TSO (The Stationery Office).

Donaldson, A. & Marshall, L. A. (2005) *Domestic Abuse Prevalence: Argyll and Clyde DAP Study*. West Dunbartonshire Domestic Abuse Partnership.

Dutton, M. A. (1992) *Empowering and Healing the Battered Woman: A Model for Assessment and Intervention*. Springer.

Feder, G., Foster, G., Eldridge, S., *et al* (2005) *Prevention of Domestic Violence (PreDoVe): A Pilot Randomised Controlled Trial of a Primary Care Based Intervention in Primary Care (Report to the Nuffield Foundation)*. Queen Mary University of London.

Feder, G., Hutson, M., Ramsay, J., *et al* (2006) Women exposed to intimate partner violence. Expectations and experiences when they encounter health-care professionals: a meta-analysis of qualitative studies. *Annals of Internal Medicine*, **166**, 22–37.

Feder, G., Agnew-Davies, R., Baird, K., *et al* (2011) Identification and Referral to Improve Safety (IRIS) of women experiencing domestic violence with a primary care training and support programme: a cluster randomised controlled trial. *Lancet*, **11**, 1–8.

Hegarty, K. (2005) What is intimate partner abuse and how common is it? In *Intimate Partner Abuse and Health Professionals: New Approaches to Domestic Violence* (eds G. Roberts, K. Hegarty & G. Feder), pp. 21–40. Elsevier.

Herman, J. L. (1998) *Trauma and Recovery: From Domestic Abuse to Political Terror*. Pandora.

James-Hanman, D. (1998) Domestic violence: breaking the silence. *Community Practitioner*, **71**, 404–407.

McNutt, L. A., Carlsen, B. E., Gagen, D., *et al* (1999) Reproductive violence screening in primary care: perspectives and experiences of patients and battered women. *Journal of the American Women's Medical Association*, **54**, 85–90.

Richards, L. (2006) Homicide prevention: findings from the Multi-agency Domestic Violence Homicide Review. *Journal of Homicide and Major Incident Investigation*, **2**, 53–72.

Richards, L., Letchford, S. & Stratton, S. (2008) *Policing Domestic Violence*. Oxford University Press.

Rodriguez, M. A., Szkupinski Quiroga, S. & Bauer, H. M. (1996) Breaking the silence: battered women's perspectives on medical care. *Archives of Family Medicine*, **5**, 153–158.

Rose, D., Trevillion, K., Woodall, A., *et al* (2011) Barriers and facilitators of disclosures of domestic violence by mental health service users: qualitative study. *British Journal of Psychiatry*, **198**, 189–194.

Stobart, E. (2009) *Multi-Agency Practice Guidelines: Handling Cases of Forced Marriage*. Foreign and Commonwealth Office, Forced Marriage Unit.

Trevillion, K., Howard, L. M., Morgan, C., *et al* (2012) The response of mental health services to domestic violence: a qualitative study of service users' and professionals' experiences. *Journal of the American Psychiatric Nurses Association*, epub ahead of print, doi: 10.1177/1078390312459747.

Walby, S. & Myhill, A. (2000) *Assessing and Managing the Risk of Domestic Violence: A Briefing Note*. Crime Reduction Research Series. Policing and Reducing Crime Unit, Home Office.

Zimmerman, C., Hossain, M., Yun, K., *et al* (2006) *Stolen Smiles: The Physical and Psychological Health Consequences of Women and Adolescents Trafficked in Europe*. London School of Hygiene and Tropical Medicine.

CHAPTER 5

Interventions for mental health service users who experience domestic violence

Kylee Trevillion and Roxane Agnew-Davies

The current evidence base on interventions to support mental health service users who experience domestic violence is limited. Three systematic reviews have examined the evidence on the effectiveness of interventions in improving mental health outcomes and safety for victims in community and healthcare settings (Ramsay *et al*, 2002, 2009; World Health Organization & London School of Hygiene and Tropical Medicine, 2010). Existing interventions include individual and group psychological therapies, psychosocial support and advocacy programmes. The methodological quality of many of these studies, however, is low (owing to small sample sizes, lack of randomised controlled trial evidence, etc. – see Feder *et al* (2009) for details) and this limits the strength of evidence for these interventions. We summarise the more robust evidence, suggest good clinical practice based on our clinical experience and the international literature, and then provide recommendations on referral pathways for clinicians following patient disclosures of domestic violence victimisation. Although there is no reason to think that victims of domestic violence who have mental disorders will not benefit from evidence-based interventions for those disorders, clinical interventions may not be as effective if domestic violence is not addressed. There is a striking lack of evidence on this issue, so this chapter focuses on the evidence for psychiatric interventions that do also address domestic violence.

Psychological interventions

Evidence-based psychological interventions should be implemented within care planning. However, well-evidenced interventions such as cognitive–behavioural therapy (CBT) and lower intensity interventions including guided self-help seem unlikely to improve outcomes for mental health patients with a history of domestic violence unless they address the abuse experienced, both by assessing risk and promoting patient safety, but also by direct acknowledgement of the psychological impact of abuse in the therapy itself. More research is needed to help guide psychological treatments for victims of violence (Nicolaidis, 2011), but clearly, therapists need to ask about and explore the acute and chronic effects of violence on their patients. It is worth remembering that the formation and maintenance of a therapeutic relationship will be more complex and subjected to greater challenges than usual if the patient is or has been a victim of domestic violence (Wilson & Lindy, 1994; Turner *et al*, 1996; Herman, 1998), because the interpersonal aspects of the trauma, such as mistrust, betrayal, dependency, love and hate tend to be replayed within the therapeutic dyad.

A wide range of individual psychological interventions has been shown to benefit female victims of domestic violence with depression and post-traumatic stress disorder (PTSD), by both reducing symptom clusters and improving self-esteem (Feder *et al*, 2009). Although most studies are of poor quality, the better-quality studies suggest that CBT for women with PTSD who are no longer experiencing violence is associated with significant improvements in symptoms of PTSD, depression and self-esteem (Feder *et al*, 2009). Such CBT programmes include feminist-oriented modules on self-advocacy and empowerment strategies (e.g. assertive communication and skills training).

Alongside individual therapeutic interventions, studies have evaluated the effectiveness of group psychological interventions and report improvements in psychological outcomes, although again these studies have major methodological limitations (Feder *et al*, 2009). The effectiveness of group interventions is therefore currently unclear. Moreover, current evidence on the effectiveness of individual and group psychological interventions cannot be extrapolated to women still in abusive relationships, or those with more severe psychiatric illnesses in contact with mental health services.

Psychological interventions in non-mental health settings

An innovative randomised controlled trial recently reported on the efficacy of an integrated multiple-risk intervention programme (targeting cigarette smoking, depression and intimate partner violence) among 913 pregnant women (El-Mohandes *et al*, 2008). The authors developed a CBT programme for depression and smoking cessation, and an individualised counselling programme for domestic violence, delivered over a minimum of four sessions prenatally and up to two sessions postpartum. The domestic violence therapeutic component was based on feminist empowerment theory; it provided information about the types of abuse and included a danger assessment component and tools for the development of a safety plan. Between baseline and postpartum follow-up, reductions in depression (from 82.7 to 54.8%) and intimate partner violence (from 50.7 to 27.3%) were reported among the intervention group, but these improvements were not statistically significant. It is likely that a more intensive intervention may be necessary to improve such complex multiple problems.

Psychological interventions in mental health settings

We are aware of only one, small randomised controlled trial of trauma-focused CBT for patients with severe mental illness. The authors (Mueser *et al*, 2008) developed a 21-week group therapy programme for men and women, which was delivered within a community mental health centre and included components such as orientation, breathing retraining, education about PTSD, cognitive restructuring, coping skills and recovery plans. Out of a total of 80 patients, 40 (59%) completed the programme (attending 11 or more sessions) and reported significant post-treatment and follow-up improvements in PTSD symptoms and diagnosis, depression and trauma-related cognitions. Those who did not complete the programme reported no significant changes in PTSD or depressive symptoms at 3 months' follow-up. These findings suggest the potential effectiveness for trauma-focused CBT in improving health outcomes among patients with a primary diagnosis of schizophrenia or major mood disorders and comorbid PTSD. However, this intervention did not specifically focus on trauma as a function of domestic violence nor on the risk of future victimisation, and longer-term follow-up data were missing.

Psychological interventions for victims of sexual assault

There are few studies to date evaluating therapeutic interventions for victims of sexual assault. Existing intervention studies – including cognitive processing therapy, stress inoculation therapy and eye movement desensitisation and reprocessing (EMDR) – have been shown to improve symptoms of PTSD among victims, although these studies often have high attrition at follow-up and do not adequately control for confounding factors. Furthermore, studies often exclude people with severe mental illness and psychiatric comorbidity, and individuals who have experienced or are currently experiencing domestic violence. It is worth noting that although there is an extensive overlap between experiences of domestic violence and sexual violence, there is a gap in research where this should be addressed.

A medical or sociopolitical issue? Service users' perspectives

It is clear from this research literature that there is a very limited evidence base on the effectiveness of psychological interventions for victims of domestic violence with mental illness. Many victims with mental health symptoms are likely to be treated with psychological interventions that do not directly address the violence. Moreover, the whole concept of offering victims of domestic violence psychological or psychiatric treatment has created considerable (and sometimes heated) debate in the past three decades. It has been argued that individual therapy by its very nature pathologises the victim, makes the abuser(s) invisible and medicalises a sociopolitical issue concerned with gender and power. It is relatively recently, in the past decade, that domestic violence services have acknowledged the value of therapy in light of a shared understanding that domestic violence does not just cause physical injury but also psychological harm, and indeed many women report that the most damaging and long-lasting effects of domestic violence are to their mental health, confidence and self-esteem (Siddiqui & Patel, 2010). One service user remarked, 'I call it symptoms of abuse' (Humphreys & Thiara, 2003).

A number of practices within the traditional medical model have also been seen as unhelpful by service users (Humphreys & Thiara, 2003). These include the lack of recognition of trauma or failure to provide trauma services; making the abuser invisible by focusing exclusively on the mental health of the victim; blaming the victim for the abuse or her reaction; offering medication rather than counselling; and the negative effects of a psychiatric diagnosis on childcare or child contact proceedings. In contrast, women identify interventions as helpful when they are encouraged to name domestic violence, are directly asked about their experiences of abuse, helped with safety planning or parenting and offered support to recover from their experiences (Humphreys & Thiara, 2003).

Domestic violence advocacy

There is growing evidence on the effectiveness of domestic violence advocacy in reducing partner violence among women who have actively sought help or are in a refuge or shelter (Feder et al, 2009). These findings support those of a previous Cochrane review of randomised controlled trials of domestic violence advocacy, which concluded that intensive advocacy (12 hours or more) may decrease physical abuse and improve quality of life, whereas brief advocacy (of less than 12 hours) may increase the use of safety behaviours among victims (Ramsay et al, 2009).

Domestic violence advocacy interventions are delivered by advocates whose core role is to provide victims with practical and emotional support; carry out risk assessments and support safety planning; provide information on welfare rights, housing options and legal issues; and signpost victims to other agencies, often advocating and working in partnership on their behalf. Several advocacy interventions are based around the concept of empowerment, which aims to help victims make sense of their experiences of abuse and responses to it; and supports them towards achieving their goals. An evaluation of the effects of advocacy in over 2000 cases across the UK found reductions in reports of severity and frequency of violence (Howarth et al, 2009), correlated with the intensity of advocacy support and number of interventions, highlighting the value of inter-agency work. However, follow-up was limited to case closure or 4 months after engagement in the service, and information on outcomes for 40% of victims who did not engage or dropped out was not available.

Domestic violence advocacy interventions in non-mental health settings

An increasing number of domestic violence advocacy interventions are being developed and evaluated within community and primary care settings, with a view to improving health and quality of life outcomes for women experiencing abuse. A systematic review of this literature found that domestic violence advocacy in community and primary care settings can reduce women's experience of abuse, increase social support and quality of life, and lead to improved use of safety behaviours and access to community resources (Feder *et al*, 2009). For example, a randomised controlled trial of domestic violence advocacy for 110 pregnant women accessing an urban public antenatal hospital and currently in an abusive relationship reported significantly less abuse and better physical functioning at follow-up among women allocated to the intervention. However, no differences were observed between intervention and control groups on general health and mental health outcomes (Tiwari *et al*, 2005). A parallel group intervention of 132 women attending a US antenatal clinic found that women receiving brief sessions of domestic violence advocacy reported significantly greater use of resources, improved safety behaviours and reductions in abuse at follow-up when compared with controls (McFarlane *et al*, 1998).

Within an accident and emergency clinic, a before-and-after study of domestic violence advocacy identified a significant increase in women's use of refuge and counselling-based services post-intervention (Feighny & Muelleman, 1999). Similarly, a UK study, published since the Feder *et al* 2009 review, conducted an evaluation of a domestic violence intervention in maternity and sexual health services. The intervention comprised guidelines and clinical training for staff, the introduction of routine enquiry about domestic violence for all patients and referral for women disclosing abuse to an on-site advocacy service. Findings suggest domestic violence training improved professionals' knowledge about domestic violence and led to positive improvements in outcomes of women accessing the advocacy services (Bacchus *et al*, 2010).

The most rigorous study of domestic violence advocacy in a healthcare setting is a recently published cluster randomised controlled trial of identification and referral to advocacy set in 51 general practices in England (Feder *et al*, 2011). The intervention programme included practice-based training sessions, a prompt within the medical record to ask about abuse and a referral pathway to a named domestic violence advocate, who also delivered the training and further consultancy. One year after the second training session, the 24 intervention practices recorded 223 referrals of patients to advocacy and the 24 control practices recorded 12 referrals (adjusted intervention rate ratio 22:1); intervention practices recorded 641 disclosures of domestic violence and control practices recorded 236 (adjusted intervention rate ratio 3:1). This trial demonstrates that such interventions in primary care can improve detection and referrals to specialist domestic violence advocates. However, it did not measure mental health outcomes for individual women referred.

Domestic violence advocacy interventions in mental health settings

To our knowledge, only one study of domestic violence advocacy has been conducted in mental health services. In this UK pilot (data available from the authors on request), we developed an advocacy intervention to support community mental health team service users who had experienced domestic violence in the previous year. The intervention consisted of reciprocal training by mental healthcare professionals and domestic violence advocates who attended interactive training sessions designed to educate each sector about the other, with a manual resource for mental healthcare professionals and regular attendance of advocates at team meetings. Clear referral pathways were developed to the advocates who provided practical and emotional support to service users (i.e. conducting risk assessments and safety plans, assisting with housing and resettlement, legal proceedings and referrals to key agencies). We found evidence to suggest that domestic violence advocacy significantly improved professionals' knowledge about domestic violence, significantly reduced abuse and improved the quality of life among victims. The nature and size of the study (the sample comprised 27 patients) limits generalisation, but this model of partnership working is promoted as good practice by UK and international guidelines (NHS Taskforce, 2010; World Health Organization, 2013). Joint working practices between mental health and domestic violence services can address both the mental health and trauma needs of victims of violence. Examples of such collaborations include representatives from both sectors participating in Multi-Agency Risk Assessment Conferences (MARACs), whereby numerous statutory and voluntary services collaborate to plan individually tailored support to protect victims at high risk of harm.

In summary, evaluations of advocacy programmes suggest that they can be effective in improving health and quality of life outcomes and reducing future victimisation, but there is little evidence on male victims of domestic violence or those diagnosed with and/or currently experiencing severe mental illness. There is still insufficient evidence for the effectiveness of domestic violence advocacy in improving mental health outcomes for victims in mental health services (Feder et al, 2009).

A caveat on using couple or family therapy if there is current domestic violence

We also need to highlight the potential dangers of couple or family-based intervention in families where there is domestic violence. Women may ask whether the partner can attend sessions, either because the partner has insisted or because the patient hopes he can be helped to change. It is also of note that 50 to 70% of couples presenting for psychological support report aggression in their relationship (Cascardi *et al*, 1992), and many couples admit to at least some history of domestic violence. If there is any indication of current domestic violence, the individuals should be offered separate therapy, even if they request conjoint work. This is because there are inherent dangers to non-abusive partners or children in couples' counselling or family therapy, which might include the therapist being unable to detect subtle signs of abuse, the risk of unwitting collusion with the perpetrator's threats, victim-blaming or minimisation and the risk that if a victim is frank about her experiences, it increases the risk to her own or the children's safety.

Many women say that they were too afraid to speak openly to therapists in the presence of the abuser; others say that their partner attended only to ensure that they did not disclose, and had threatened consequences if they did. Others, who did have the courage to speak within the apparent safety of the therapist's office, have been punished later by abuse at home; consequently, women quickly learn not to speak within the session, or the couple drop out of therapy. The violence of the abuser (the real source of trauma) can be masked behind a focus on communication, parenting or family relationships. Moreover, joint counselling can imply that a victim has joint responsibility for the violence and for making it stop. The evidence is that couple therapy is not only ineffective but that it increases the risk of harm to the woman (Galvani, 2007; Tunariu, 2007). In the UK, Relate has piloted and rolled out an assessment and treatment protocol to ensure that when domestic violence is disclosed, individual therapy preceded any couple work (Tunariu, 2007).

It is important for healthcare practitioners to develop strategies to manage situations where abusers are present during clinical assessments. The following steps can be used in these instances:

1   Communicate concerns about the 'conflict'.
2   Reinforce that your role as therapist is to ensure everyone feels safe and is able to talk openly.
3   Inform them that the next routine step is to talk to each person alone.
4   Reassure them that you are not withdrawing support and want to fully understand each person's perspective.
5   State you are pleased that the issue has been raised – this shows open communication, willingness to talk about difficult issues and a commitment to promote the well-being of the couple or family.
6   Talk separately with each person about your concerns and their views on what should happen next.
7   Offer specialist information and referral opportunities.
8   Consider child protection issues and potential referrals to safeguard the children.

Referrals for perpetrators can include referral to specialist agencies (e.g. Respect, www.respect.uk.net). There has been increasing awareness that anger is not a key factor in understanding or intervening to reduce domestic violence. Programmes based on anger management can reinforce beliefs that justify abuse of power and control and there are inherent dangers in overlooking coercive, controlling behaviours (Stark, 2007; Tunariu, 2007).

Good practice recommendations for mental health services in responding to domestic violence

As highlighted in Chapter 2, mental health service users are at increased risk of violence and as a consequence are particularly vulnerable to re-victimisation, including for domestic violence but also for other forms of violence. Therefore, it is important for mental health services to ensure professionals are aware of this risk and formulate risk assessments and care plans that incorporate interventions to address issues of safety and risk of future victimisation. This section outlines existing interventions that can be effective in preventing re-victimisation, promoting safety and improving outcomes for service users disclosing domestic violence. In addition, Box 5.1 (p. 75) outlines examples of good practice.

Multi-Agency Risk Assessment Conferences (MARACs)

MARACs were first introduced in England and Wales in April 2003. They are multi-agency meetings between statutory and voluntary sector organisations who share information about domestic violence victims at high risk of harm and develop coordinated action plans to increase their safety (Home Office, 2011). The organisations that attend each MARAC vary but usually include representation from police and probation services, independent domestic violence advisors, children's services and health and housing representatives.

There are approximately 250 MARACs currently operating in England and Wales, with the majority of meetings occurring at least monthly (Home Office Violent and Youth Crime Prevention Unit & Research and Analysis Unit, 2011). Between 2010 and 2011, 242 MARACs supported 49 819 adult cases and 65 842 associated children's cases (linked to the adult victims) in total. The MARAC meetings aim to:
- increase the safety, health and well-being of victims and their children through inter-agency information-sharing;
- determine whether the alleged perpetrator poses a significant risk to any particular individual or to the general community;
- provide professional support to all those at risk and reduce repeat victimisation through the construction and implementation of coordinated safety plans;

- offer specialist support to the victim which is independent of the criminal justice system through the independent domestic violence advisor role;
- improve inter-agency accountability.

Evidence on the effectiveness of MARACs

One of the first evaluations of MARACs examined the number of police complaints and police call-outs for domestic violence at 6 and 12 months after a MARAC had been initiated and found that they were effective in reducing the risk of harm among victims (Robinson, 2004), recorded by both police call-outs and interviews with victims. A literature review of the effectiveness of MARACs identified that this intervention can help to improve victim safety and reduce re-victimisation (Home Office Violent and Youth Crime Prevention Unit & Research and Analysis Unit, 2011). These findings are particularly notable given the extensive histories of harm and the high risk of repeated violence among victims referred to MARACs. However, a report on four London MARACs unveiled some variations in styles and efficacy across MARACs in different areas as they evolve, including their regard for victim consent, threshold of risk for inclusion, perspectives on domestic violence, reviews of cases and action plans, the quality of contributions, and seniority of attendance by representatives from different agencies, including mental health services (Coy & Kelly, 2011). A cost–benefit analysis of MARAC services estimated that for every £1 spent on MARACs, at least £6 of public money can be saved annually on direct costs to agencies such as the police and health services, potentially saving £740 million (Co-ordinated Action Against Domestic Abuse, 2010).

Mental health services representation at MARACs

Specific guidance for mental health professionals on the process of local MARACs and how to refer service users can be accessed through local domestic violence coordinators or local domestic violence agencies. The national charity Co-ordinated Action Against Domestic Abuse (CAADA) prepared a toolkit on training, guidance, policy and data insight to support professionals and organisations working with victims of domestic abuse (www.caada.org.uk). The guidance includes a risk identification checklist for clinicians to pinpoint those service users who are at increased risk of harm (Appendix 1).

Although most relevant professionals believe mental health services should be represented at MARACs, currently only 34% of MARACs have a mental health professional consistently attend, and it is notable that some of the barriers to effective MARAC working are the lack of referrals from or participation by non-police agencies including mental health services (Coy & Kelly, 2011; Home Office Violent and Youth Crime Prevention Unit & Research and Analysis Unit, 2011). Indeed, as many of the cases seen at MARACs involve mental health issues, either for the victim, the perpetrator or both, the involvement of mental health services is essential to ensure the efficacy of a safety plan.

Domestic violence services

The free-phone 24-hour National Domestic Violence Helpline (0808 2000 247) run by Refuge in partnership with Women's Aid can advise on local domestic violence services, as well as offering direct support to women callers. Local domestic services across the country offer independent advocacy, advice and outreach services to women in the local community. Refuges are safe houses for women and children who are fleeing domestic violence. They provide safe and emergency accommodation and independent domestic violence advocacy for women. Many refuges have resources to support women with a physical disability; some offer individual counselling or group sessions and some have support services for children.

Domestic violence services for victims from minority ethnic groups

There are over 500 refuge and support services in England, Scotland, Wales and Northern Ireland, with some offering specialist services for women of particular ethnic or cultural backgrounds (Appendix 2). In 2009, the Home Office funded a pilot programme, 'the Sojourner project', to provide support for abused women with no recourse to public funds who came to the UK on a spousal visa. This project sought to assist abused women without indefinite leave to remain by providing refuges with 4 weeks (20 working days) of funding to cover victims' housing and living costs. During this time, women were encouraged to complete an application for indefinite leave to remain under the domestic violence rule and once this application was submitted to the UK Border Agency, funding was provided to the refuge for a maximum of 4 additional weeks (20 working days) while the UK Border Agency considered the application. If the UK Border Agency approved this application, the victim was allowed to remain in the UK. Following the results of this pilot, the UK Border Agency introduced the Destitution Domestic Violence (DDV) concession, which allows victims of domestic violence with no recourse to public funds to access public resources for a period of 3 months while they make a claim for indefinite leave to remain (UK Border Agency, 2012).

Domestic violence services for victims with mental illness/substance misuse problems

A handful of UK refuges have established specialist provision to support the needs of women with a mental illness and/or problematic substance use (e.g. by extending staff cover out of hours and active efforts to collaborate with local specialist drug and alcohol teams). However, supporting the needs of mentally ill women poses a challenge to many mainstream domestic violence and refuge services, who have had little training and feel ill equipped to provide the support of the nature, intensity and quality required. Thus in the UK and internationally, and despite the efforts of Women's Aid to reduce the exclusion of mentally ill women from access to mainstream services since 2005, women with severe mental disorders may find it difficult to access refuges (Howard *et al*, 2010). Often, by the time they access domestic violence services, they have become trapped in situations that exacerbate their social exclusion, sometimes paraphrased as 'chaotic lives', and thereby encounter difficulties in sustaining tenancies and living within a structured environment (Hager, 2011).

Referral pathways following disclosures of domestic violence

We recommend developing close working and strategic partnership arrangements with local domestic violence outreach or refuge services so that both sectors understand which services the other sector can provide for victims of domestic violence with mental health problems. An effective local model of collaboration will specify the roles of each agency as well as stress the importance of and outline opportunities for inter-agency contributions and review on a case-led basis. Although historically these sectors have diverged in their philosophical approach and service provision, integrated service strategies are badly needed to prevent women with complex needs being excluded from services. Services also need to ensure that professionals are aware that individuals with mental disorder (particularly those with serious mental disorder) are vulnerable to future victimisation (including domestic violence) and that in addition to addressing current experiences, professionals need to address this vulnerability in risk formulations and interventions.

Previous experience on developing these integrated services suggests that the first steps in developing a specialist, integrated service is, where possible, to involve individuals with experience in each of the specialist fields (i.e. domestic violence, substance misuse treatment, mental health services and intellectual disabilities) and/or to give all staff comprehensive training on the multiple issues, their assessment and effective responses to specific needs (Nosek & Howland, 1998; Najavits, 2002; Zweig *et al*, 2002). Second, the staff need to work together to understand one another's approaches and treatment strategies, to develop trust and respect and to build a consensus on how best to integrate the services. Collaboration with other agencies focusing specifically on the additional barrier/barriers faced by women is the third key to the successful implementation of integrated strategies. In other words, mental health services cannot do it alone. Taking the time to develop trust and consensus among partner agencies is the best way to build well-functioning coordinated responses to violence against women who are challenged by multiple barriers.

It has also been suggested that:

- barriers to services should be eliminated by providing clear information and referral services;
- the physical accessibility of facilities should be ensured (that may include 24-hour access to transportation);
- there should be provision for interpreters, care assistants or communication assistance;
- staff should be trained to monitor risks and plan effective responses;
- victims who are dependent on caregivers may need special legal protection against abuse.

Lessons learnt from international specialist providers

Zweig *et al* (2002) asked integrated specialist services about lessons learnt while implementing programmes to serve women with complex needs. The advice offered is listed in Box 5.1.

Conclusions

The evidence base on interventions for domestic violence is limited, but there is growing evidence for the effectiveness of intervention packages which include training of healthcare professionals, with domestic violence

---

Box 5.1   Advice to professionals helping abused women with complex needs

- Be patient and persistent – change is a long process. Women with multiple issues require more time from service providers than women who do not have multiple issues.
- Establishing collaborations with other agencies and working with different people is a major key to success. Providing your service alone will not work.
- Work to have all levels of agencies committed to the joint work and knowledgeable about the issues of interest.
- Concurrently address the many problems women face because the issues, such as violence and problematic substance use, are all connected.
- Provide services to the clients wherever they are, meaning both the physical location and their readiness for services.
- Offer trust, respect and compassion; look beyond the problem or behaviour to see the person.
- Do not expect or insist on consistency from clients.
- Tread lightly when working with other service providers so you do not alienate them; start where they need to start and recognise that you may need to educate them around issues of multiple barriers and about victims of violence.
- Language is important, for example talk about women who have experienced domestic violence and who also have problematic substance use rather than 'mentally ill, alcoholic women'.

---

advocacy as a clear option in a referral and care pathway. In addition, although the evidence on psychological interventions is limited, it is clear that the trauma experienced by victims needs to be addressed in therapy which can then lead to improvements in psychological symptoms and social functioning. Good practice guidelines emphasise the need for partnership work with local domestic violence services as well as other agencies and stress that safeguarding vulnerable adults and children requires better mental health representation at MARACs.

References

Bacchus, L. J., Bewley, S., Torres Vitolas, C., *et al* (2010) Evaluation of a domestic violence intervention in the maternity and sexual health services of a UK hospital. *Reproductive Health Matters*, **18**, 147–157.

Cascardi, M., Langhinrichsen, J. & Vivian, D. (1992) Marital aggression: impact, injury, and health correlates for husbands and wives. *Archives of Internal Medicine*, **152**, 1178–1184.

Co-ordinated Action Against Domestic Abuse (2010) *Saving Lives, Saving Money: MARACs and High Risk Domestic Abuse*. CAADA.

Coy, M. & Kelly, L. (2011) *Islands in the Stream: An Evaluation of Four London Independent Domestic Violence Advocacy Schemes*. London Metropolitan University, Child and Woman Abuse Studies Unit.

El-Mohandes, A. A. E., Kiely, M., Joseph, J. G., *et al* (2008) An intervention to improve postpartum outcomes in African–American mothers: a randomized controlled trial. *Obstetrics & Gynecology*, **112**, 611–620.

Feder, G., Ramsay, J., Dunne, D., *et al* (2009) How far does screening women for domestic (partner) violence in different health-care settings meet criteria for a screening programme? Systematic reviews of nine UK National Screening Committee critieria. *Health Technology Assessment*, **13**, iii–113.

Feder, G., Agnew-Davies, R., Baird, K., *et al* (2011) Identification and Referral to Improve Safety (IRIS) of women experiencing domestic violence with a primary care training and support programme: a cluster randomised controlled trial. *Lancet*, **11**, 1–8.

Feighny, K. M. & Muelleman, R. L. (1999) The effect of a community-based intimate partner violence advocacy program in the emergency department on identification rate of intimate partner violence. *Missouri Medicine*, **96**, 242–244.

Galvani, S. (2007) Safety in numbers? Tackling domestic abuse in couples and network therapies. *Drug and Alcohol Review*, **26**, 175–181.

Hager, D. (2011) *Finding Safety. Provision of Specialised Domestic Violence and Refuge Services for Women who Currently Find it Difficult to Access Mainstream Services: Disabled Women, Older Women, Sex Workers and Women with Mental Illness and/or Drug and Alcohol Problems as a Result of Domestic Violence*. Winston Churchill Memorial Trust.

Herman, J. L. (1998) *Trauma and Recovery: From Domestic Abuse to Political Terror*. Pandora.

Home Office (2011) *Call to End Violence Against Women and Girls: Action Plan Progress Review*. Home Office.

Home Office Violent and Youth Crime Prevention Unit & Research and Analysis Unit (2011) *Research into Multi-Agency Risk Assessment Conferences (MARACs)*. Home Office.

Howard, L. M., Trevillion, K. & Agnew-Davies, R. (2010) Domestic violence and mental health. *International Review of Psychiatry*, **22**, 525–534.

Howarth, E., Stimpson, L., Barran, D., *et al* (2009) *Safety in Numbers: A Multi-Site Evaluation of Independent Domestic Violence Advocacy Services*. The Henry Smith Charity.

Humphreys, C. & Thiara, R. (2003) Mental health and domestic violence: 'I call it symptoms of abuse'. *British Journal of Social Work*, **33**, 209–226.

McFarlane, J., Parker, B., Soeken, K., *et al* (1998) Safety behaviors of abused women after an intervention during pregnancy. *Journal of Obstetric, Gynecologic and Neonatal Nursing*, **27**, 64–69.

Mueser, K. T., Rosenberg, S. D., Xie, H., *et al* (2008) A randomized controlled trial of cognitive-behavioral treatment for posttraumatic stress disorder in severe mental illness. *Journal of Consulting and Clinical Psychology*, **76**, 259–271.

Najavits, L. M. (2002) *Seeking Safety: A Treatment Manual for PTSD and Substance Abuse.* Guilford Press.

NHS Taskforce (2010) *Responding to Violence against Women and Children – The Role of the NHS (Report from the Domestic Violence Sub-Group).* Department of Health.

Nicolaidis, C. (2011) Violence and poor mental health and functional outcomes. *BMJ*, **343**, d7311.

Nosek, M. A. & Howland, C. A. (1998) Abuse and women with disabilities. *VAWnet Applied Research Forum*, 1–**5**.

Ramsay, J., Richardson, J., Carter, Y. H., *et al* (2002) Should health professionals screen for domestic violence? Systematic review. *BMJ*, **325**, 1–13.

Ramsay, J., Carter, Y., Davidson, L., *et al* (2009) Advocacy interventions to reduce or eliminate violence and promote the physical and psychosocial well-being of women who experience intimate partner abuse. *Cochrane Database of Systematic Reviews*, **3**, CD005043.

Robinson, A. L. (2004) *Domestic Violence MARACs (Multi-Agency Risk Assessment Conferences) for Very High-Risk Victims in Cardiff, Wales: A Process and Outcome Evaluation.* Cardiff University.

Siddiqui, H. & Patel, M. (2010) *Safe and Sane: A Model of Intervention on Domestic Violence and Mental Health, Suicide and Self-Harm Amongst Black and Minority Ethnic Women.* Southall Black Sisters.

Stark, E. (2007) *Coercive Control: How Men Entrap Women in Personal Life.* Oxford University Press.

Tiwari, A., Leung, W. C., Leung, T. W., *et al* (2005) A randomised controlled trial of empowerment training for Chinese abused pregnant women in Hong Kong. *BJOG: An International Journal of Obstetrics & Gynaecology*, **112**, 1249–1256.

Tunariu, A. D. (2007) *Bridging to Change: Expanding Relate's Capacity to Provide Work with Clients Who Use Domestic Violence and Abuse and to Meet the Needs of Clients Whose Lives are Affected by It. A Review of Three Domestic Violence and Abuse Prevention Programmes (DVA-PP).* Relate.

Turner, S. W., McFarlane, A. C. & van der Kolk, B. A. (1996) The therapeutic environment and new explorations in the treatment of post traumatic stress disorder. In *Traumatic Stress: The Effects of Overwhelming Experience on Mind, Body and Society* (eds B. A. van der Kolk, A. C. McFarlane & L. Weisaeth), pp. 537–558. Guilford Press.

UK Border Agency (2012) *Protecting Victims of Domestic Violence: A New Immigration Policy.* UK Border Agency.

Wilson, J. P. & Lindy, J. D. (eds) (1994) *Countertransference in the Treatment of PTSD.* Guilford Press.

World Health Organization (2013) *Guideline Development Group on Policy and Clinical Practice Guidelines for Responding to Violence Against Women (2011–2012).* WHO (in press).

World Health Organization & London School of Hygiene and Tropical Medicine (2010) *Preventing Intimate Partner and Sexual Violence against Women: Taking Action and Generating Evidence.* WHO.

Zweig, J. M., Schlichter, K. A. & Burt, M. R. (2002) Assisting women victims of violence who experience multiple barriers to services. *Violence Against Women*, **8**, 162–180.

Resources

Further details about UK-wide domestic violence services can be found at www. womensaid.org.uk and in Appendix 2.

CHAPTER 6

Medico-legal issues

Fiona Mason

There are many areas of overlap between psychiatry and the law in the field of domestic violence. Mental health professionals need to be aware of their statutory and professional responsibilities, and criminal and civil court processes, given the possibility that they may be called to give evidence.

This chapter outlines key elements of this medico-legal interface; it focuses on the law as it currently stands in England and Wales, although many of the principles outlined are similar to those in other jurisdictions.

Safeguarding vulnerable adults

Safeguarding is about the well-being of adults who may have difficulty in protecting themselves from harm and abuse and in promoting their own interests. All persons have the right to live their lives free from violence and abuse. *Safeguarding Adults* (Association of Directors of Social Services, 2005) recognises the changing context from providing protection to promoting active citizenship. It replaces a narrower focus on the protection of 'vulnerable' adults and now encompasses all work which enables an adult 'who is or may be eligible for community care services' (Lord Chancellor's Department, 1997) to retain independence, well-being and choice, and to access their right to live free from abuse and neglect.

The overlap between safeguarding adults and domestic violence is significant, not least because domestic violence in itself can have a significant impact on mental health, as discussed in Chapter 2. This in turn may result in the victim becoming a vulnerable adult. There is also evidence that domestic violence is perpetrated disproportionately against vulnerable groups. Women who use mental health services are much more likely to have experienced domestic violence than women in the general population, and many older women also experience domestic violence (O'Keefe *et al*, 2007). Women with disabilities are also particularly vulnerable to abuse (Brownridge, 2006). Safeguarding arrangements are therefore not only often applicable, but highly relevant to these vulnerable populations. It is of note that a recent study found that professionals working within mental health services in the UK were not clear about referral pathways for those experiencing domestic violence, and expressed mixed views on the value of vulnerable adult procedures (Trevillion *et al*, 2012). It is therefore vital that services strive to ensure that there is joined-up thinking and practice across the disciplines, given that significant numbers of victims of domestic violence are vulnerable adults and *vice versa*.

Definitions used in this chapter:

(a)   adult – anyone aged 18 years and over;

(b)   vulnerable – anyone who is, or may be, in need of community services by reason of mental health or other disabilities, age or illness, and who is unable to take care of themselves or protect themselves against harm or exploitation (Department of Health, 2000); a clear distinction must be made between those who have capacity and those who have impaired capacity or who lost their capacity; a key factor in assessing vulnerability is an individual's ability to protect themselves or promote their own interests;

(c)   abuse – any act (such as domestic violence) which causes harm to another.

Capacity and consent

Decision-making in relation to adults who lack capacity is regulated in England and Wales by the Mental Capacity Act 2005, in Scotland by the Adults with Incapacity (Scotland) Act 2000 and in Northern Ireland by the common law. Where a vulnerable adult does not have capacity or where a serious allegation has been made and the vulnerable adult does not wish to make a complaint, those responsible for their care have an obligation to act on their behalf. Thus it may be necessary for professionals to override confidentiality to ensure the vulnerable adult is protected. Such decisions are clearly difficult and have to be considered on an individual basis, taking into account the level of threat presented.

Where an individual has capacity, professionals will need to respect their decision in relation to reporting safeguarding issues. However, if there are any issues relating to the protection of children or the public, professionals should involve relevant agencies.

Principles

The government's policy objective is to prevent and reduce the risk of significant harm to vulnerable adults from abuse or other types of exploitation, while supporting individuals in maintaining control over their lives and in making informed choices without coercion. At the core of the government's new policy for safeguarding vulnerable adults are six key principles that were developed for application across the health, social care and criminal justice sectors:

1   Empowerment – promotion of independence and presumption of person-led decisions and informed consent.

79

2 Protection – support and representation for those in greatest need.

3 Prevention – it is better to take action before harm occurs.

4 Proportionality – proportionate and least intrusive response appropriate to the risk presented.

5 Partnership – safeguarding is the most effective way individuals, professionals and communities work together to prevent, detect and respond to harm and abuse.

6 Transparency and accountability – there must be accountability (e.g. through clinical audit) and transparency in delivering safeguarding.

In addition to these principles, providers must avoid discriminating between differing groups of patients. Decisions made must be on the basis of fair and objective assessment of individual needs.

Procedures

Systems and procedures for protecting vulnerable adults are not yet uniform, but a number of key points apply to all health professionals who may encounter vulnerable adults. Health professionals should be able to identify adults who are vulnerable, routinely enquire about experience of violence and abuse at assessment and reviews (Department of Health, 2008), and be familiar with local procedures and protocols.

Safeguarding is everyone's business, but given the complexity of this area of practice it is recommended that a stepped approach is taken (British Medical Association, 2011).

Step one: prevention

Staff must be aware of the possibility of abuse. Practitioners should be able to identify those adults in their care who may be vulnerable and should record factors that may contribute to that vulnerability. They will then be able to ensure that the individual receives necessary support.

Step two: assessing the individual's needs

Once a vulnerable individual has been identified, their needs should be assessed. A broad assessment of vulnerability and needs is required; one which moves beyond assessing a person's ability/inability to meet their own basic needs, to investigate the full history and dynamic of the abusive relationship and to identify the factors, such as control and isolation, that are acting as barriers to self-help. Where harm or abuse has already occurred, or a person is at immediate risk, consideration should be given to whether the local authority adult safeguarding procedures should be engaged.

Step three: responding to harm or abuse – assessing competence

Where there are doubts about an individual's decision-making capacity this should be assessed. Persons with capacity have the right to make decisions about their own care and treatment whereas treatment decisions made on behalf of adults lacking capacity should be made with their best interests in mind.

Step four: responding to harm or abuse – identifying relevant services

Relevant supporting services should be identified and offered. Consideration needs to be given to the identification of services beyond direct health needs; personal and social factors should be included in any assessment of need.

Step five: responding to harm or abuse – taking a consensual approach

Where an adult with capacity declines services, reasons should be explored and alternatives offered.

Step six: safeguarding

Local measures are in place to protect those least able to protect themselves. Safeguards against harm and abuse need to be an integral part of care and support. Safeguarding procedures facilitate multiprofessional working and in case of domestic violence, input from a number of organisations will be required.

Good safeguarding arrangements should incorporate the following stages and procedures: referral, strategy meeting, investigation, protection and preservation of evidence, recording and monitoring.

Referral

From the point where someone either identifies or suspects abuse, or where abuse is reported by the vulnerable adult, the local safeguarding adults procedures must be followed. If, at any point, the situation is, or becomes, life threatening, dangerous or obviously criminal, the police must be involved immediately.

Overall responsibility for coordinating multi-agency responses to the harm or abuse of vulnerable adults rests with the local authority. Generally to refer, a notification form will be completed. The completed form must then be sent to the local adult protection team and locally identified individuals. Generally, where incidents are deemed to be a safeguarding adults incident, an urgent meeting will be called. Investigations will either be internal (the local care team meeting will often act as the strategy discussion) or external, when an appointed officer will liaise with the local organisation who should nominate an individual to attend the strategy meeting.

Strategy meeting

This is to ensure that the alleged victim is protected. Information must be shared and an investigating officer appointed. The lead officer must ensure that there is appropriate representation (i.e. all the relevant agencies are present) at all necessary meetings during the investigation. Accountability and monitoring arrangements must be clear. A review date must be set. If the police are the investigating officers, then their processes take precedence.

The attendance of the alleged victim at the meeting should always be considered and alleged perpetrators excluded from the meeting.

The investigation

The investigating officer must coordinate and collect information, although police investigations take precedence. Once the investigation is complete and the information collated, a further meeting of the strategy group should be convened. The purpose of this second meeting is to produce a safeguarding plan and clarify any further actions.

Protection and preservation of evidence

Given the criminal nature of domestic violence, it is vital that potential evidence is not destroyed. Where there is evidence of physical assault, such as bruising, photographs must be taken immediately and stored safely and securely. Where police are involved they may take photographs for their records. Any subsequent medical examinations should ideally be carried out by a suitably qualified forensic medical examiner.

Recording and monitoring

Care organisations must keep comprehensive records of any work undertaken under the safeguarding adults procedure, including all alerts and referrals made (Association of Directors of Social Services, 2005).

Role of the safeguarding adult lead: all organisations have a responsibility to designate a lead person for the implementation of *Safeguarding Adults* (National Framework Standard 2; Association of Directors of Social Services, 2005).

Further literature on safeguarding adults is available at the end of this chapter.

Safeguarding vulnerable children

Definitions:
(a) child – the Children Act 1989 and the Children Act 2004 define a child as a person up to the age of 18. The fact that a child has reached 16 years of age, is living independently or is in further education, is a member of the armed forces, is in hospital, prison or in a young offenders' institution, does not change his or her status or entitlement to services or protection under the Children Act 1989 (HM Government, 2010);
(b) child abuse – the term used when a person harms a child. A person can abuse or neglect a child by inflicting harm or failing to prevent harm to the child.

There is a strong correlation between domestic violence and child maltreatment because children may directly suffer violence themselves or they may witness it. The UK Adoption and Children Act 2002 (which came into force in 2005) extended the legal definition of harming children to include harm suffered by witnessing the ill-treatment of others, especially in the home. Living with domestic violence distorts children's perceptions of relationships, blame, cause and effect, and it has a profound impact on their cognitive, psychological, social and educational development. Over any 100-day period an estimated 205 000 children will witness domestic violence (Department of Health, 2002), and in households with children where there is domestic violence, the children witness about three-quarters of the abusive incidents (Royal College of Psychiatrists, 2013). Around half the children in such families have themselves been badly hit or beaten. Sexual and emotional abuse is also more likely to happen in families where there is violence.

The issue of children living with domestic violence is now recognised as a matter for concern in its own right by both government and key children's services agencies. The link between child physical abuse and domestic violence is high, with estimates ranging between 30 and 66%, depending on the study (Edleson, 1999; Hester *et al*, 2000; Humphreys & Thiara, 2002).

All the five key outcomes for children identified in *Every Child Matters: Change for Children* (being healthy, staying safe, enjoying and achieving, making a positive contribution, economic well-being; HM Government, 2004) can be adversely affected for a child living with domestic violence and abuse – the impact is usually on every aspect of a child's life. This will vary according to the child's resilience and the strengths and weaknesses of their particular circumstances.

The three central imperatives of any intervention for children living with domestic violence are:

1   to protect the child/children;
2   to support the victim to protect themselves and their child/children; and
3   to hold the abusive partner accountable for the violence and provide them with opportunities to change.

Safeguarding children is the responsibility of everyone. For all safeguarding issues social workers are recognised as lead professionals. The Directorate of Social Care and Health (Social Services) is legally responsible for taking immediate action on child protection issues where the child is in their area at the time of the incident or allegation. They should attempt to involve the original local authority as far as possible.

Children may be directly abused in families where domestic violence occurs, but seeing or hearing the ill treatment of another person in the context of domestic violence can also have an impact on children (see Chapter 1, pp. 12–13). The adverse effects may include:

- physical injury
- developmental delay
- low take-up of healthcare
- emotional and behavioural difficulties

- mental health difficulties
- lower educational achievements.

The specific effects of witnessing domestic violence vary for each child, according to many factors including age, stage of development, level of violence, gender, role in the family, relationship with parents and availability of outside support.

Other forms of abuse which should trigger safeguarding children procedures include:

- emotional abuse
- neglect
- sexual abuse
- child trafficking
- exploitation on the internet
- bullying, racism and other types of discrimination.

Procedures

Everyone has a responsibility to identify, protect and refer children who may be at risk. When domestic violence is reported, consideration needs to be given to the position of the child within the family. Although they may not be subject to direct violence themselves, the witnessing of violence in the family would in itself potentially constitute a safeguarding issue.

Practices and procedures should complement the responsibilities of statutory agencies in relation to child protection. Clinicians should be aware that all complaints, allegations and incidents of child abuse should be reported to children's social care services. It should never be assumed that someone else will take care of the issues arising from domestic violence. If domestic violence is disclosed, then the clinician should explain that priority will be given to ensuring that the child/children and the non-abusive parent's safety are not compromised through the sharing of information.

Clinicians should be mindful that abusers may have threatened victims that the children will be removed. Chapter 4 (e.g. pp. 51–55) suggests some ways to reassure victims that it is the abuse that is the problem and that it is not their fault. It should be noted, though, that clinicians should never give absolute guarantees of confidentiality to children or adults wishing to tell them something serious, for instance the disclosure of violence or abuse. Professionals should validate and support children who disclose, listening, taking the disclosure seriously, explaining the need to ensure safety, reassuring, and providing relevant contact details for domestic violence services and children's agencies and helplines (see Appendix 2 for contact telephone numbers and website addresses for a number of such agencies).

Whether or not a child or their parent (usually the mother) discloses, when a clinician becomes aware of domestic violence in the family, they must assess and attend to immediate safety issues and establish:

- the nature of the violence
- whether there are other children in the household
- where the offender is
- what the immediate fears are
- whether there is a need to seek immediate assistance
- whether the child/children and non-abusive parent have somewhere safe to go.

The clinician should make a decision about whether other agencies should be involved, record the information and discuss their concerns with the agency's nominated safeguarding children advisor. Local procedures should then be followed and should include a risk assessment which will help determine what further action should be taken.

The Mental Health Act and domestic violence

Offenders under the Mental Health Act

The 2007 amendments to the Mental Health Act 1983 extended (from 3 November 2008) victims' rights under the Domestic Violence, Crime and Victims Act 2004 to victims of offenders who are detained, or on supervised community treatment, as unrestricted patients under Part 3 of the Mental Health Act. As a result, hospital managers, responsible clinicians, approved mental health professionals and National Health Service (NHS) bodies that fund treatment of such patients in the independent sector have new duties.

Under the Domestic Violence, Crime and Victims Act 2004, victims of certain sexual and violent offenders have certain rights to receive information over the course of the offender's sentence and to make representations about any conditions to which the offender should be subject on release. The spirit of these changes relates to information-sharing and allowing victims to have a voice. These rights have applied since 1 July 2005 to victims of offenders who are detained in hospital under Part 3 of the Mental Health Act 1983 (the section dealing with patients concerned in criminal proceedings or under sentence) and who are subject to special restrictions (restricted patients), including those who have been conditionally discharged. From 3 November 2008, these rights were extended to victims of offenders detained in hospital under Part 3 of the Act who are not subject to special restrictions (unrestricted patients), including those who are discharged from hospital into supervised community treatment.

To enable victims to exercise those rights, there are new statutory duties on agencies responsible for managing psychiatric patients:

1 Providers of probation services – to identify eligible victims and, with their consent, to pass on their details to hospital managers.
2 Hospital managers – to give information to victims and to pass on any representations they make to the person responsible for determining the matter.

3   Responsible clinicians – to inform hospital managers if they are considering discharging relevant unrestricted patients and if they make certain decisions relating to those patients. They must also consider victims' representations when deciding what conditions to include in the community treatment order of an unrestricted patient they discharge into supervised community treatment. Where representations influence, for instance, the location for discharge or the conditions of any community treatment order (CTO), clinicians will need to consider the usual balance with Articles 5, 8 and 11 of the Human Rights Act and the European Convention on Human Rights. In terms of Article 8 (right to respect for private and family life), it was found in *L v. Sweden, App. No. 10801/84* that decisions taken are reasonable if the order is done in accordance with the law and is necessary in a democratic society. Presumably, this would equally apply if impingement of the articles was occurring as a result of the Domestic Violence, Crime and Victims Act influencing the community treatment order.

4   Approved mental health professionals – to consider victims' representations when deciding whether to agree to the proposed conditions to be included in a community treatment order for a relevant unrestricted patient being discharged into supervised community treatment.

5   NHS bodies – if they are considering using their powers under Section 23(3) of the Mental Health Act 1983 to discharge relevant NHS patients who are detained in independent hospitals, or supervised community treatment patients for whom an independent hospital is the responsible hospital.

Victims treated under the Mental Health Act

When treating victims of domestic violence under a section of the Mental Health Act, confidentiality and safety need to be carefully thought about if considering involving partners in discussions over treatment. For example, staff should not disclose information on a victim's whereabouts without ensuring it is safe to do so. Where the nearest relative is identified as an abuser, displacement should be considered on the basis that they may not be acting in the victim's best interests. In such circumstances, contact should be made with the hospital's Mental Health Act office.

Other relevant legislation

Domestic violence is a crime under both civil and criminal law.

In civil law, someone (a plaintiff) applies to a court so that their case against a defendant can be heard. Plaintiffs and defendants can be private individuals or any other single legal entity such as a company, local authority or business partnership. Civil law applies to the principles of common law, but in civil actions, unlike criminal proceedings, the Crown takes no side, although the Crown does supply the court, the judge and, if necessary, the enforcement of the judge's rulings.

Criminal law is made by the Crown, although it is drafted by government and passed by parliament before it goes to the monarch for Royal Assent. Under this law the Crown has the right to prosecute citizens for criminal offences.

Relevant legislation is summarised in the following section.

Civil action

Family Law Act 1996 Part IV

The Act provides for a single set of remedies to deal with domestic violence and to regulate occupation of the family home, through two specific types of order, the non-molestation order and the occupation order. The Act covers people who:

- are or have been married to each other;
- are cohabitants or former cohabitants (opposite gender);
- live or have lived in the same household, not just as employee, tenant, lodger or boarder;
- are relatives;
- have formally agreed to marry each other;
- are both the parents of the same child or have had parental responsibility for that child;
- are both involved in the same family proceedings (e.g. divorce, child contact).

People who do not meet these criteria might take action through the courts under the Protection from Harassment Act 1997.

Non-molestation order

This is a court order to prevent someone from using or threatening violence, or from intimidating, harassing or pestering a victim. It can have very specific instructions in it to suit particular circumstances – for example, it can order an abuser to stop texting or waiting outside a workplace. An order may be made for a specified period, usually 6 months, for an open-ended period, or until a different order is made if further provisions are needed.

Occupation order

This is an order that regulates who can live in the family home. The court has power to order someone to live only in a certain part of the house or to allow someone back into the house, etc. The court has wide powers to order someone not to surrender a tenancy or remove or destroy the contents of the home. Any person associated with the respondent may apply for an order and an application may be made on behalf of a relevant child.

If an order is awarded, it is a good idea for your patient to keep a copy of any order and any power of arrest document at home and about their person to show their local police or community safety unit and also to make sure it is registered on their computer system.

Under the Children Act 1989 there are several orders that can be useful for women and children escaping domestic violence. It is best to suggest that your patient seeks the advice of a solicitor who specialises in family law. If you or they need information, you can also access free legal advice from Rights of Women (www.rightsofwomen.org.uk; their free telephone helpline is staffed by qualified solicitors; for contact details see Appendix 2).

Women without recourse to public funds (or with limited right to remain in the country) are particularly vulnerable to exploitation. It is critical they are supported to access a reputable firm of solicitors who are specialists in immigration law.

Power of arrest

To provide better protection, the powers of arrest in relation to the non-molestation order and the occupation order have been strengthened. Under the Domestic Violence, Crime and Victims Act 2004, a breach of a non-molestation order is a criminal offence so arrest can be actioned. Where the court makes an occupation order and it appears to the court that an ex-partner has used or threatened physical violence against the individual or their child, then the court can attach a power of arrest. This means that a copy of the order must be held on record at the police station and the police can arrest the perpetrator without a warrant, immediately, if the order is broken. The police must reasonably suspect that the perpetrator breached some provisions of the order.

Court procedure and privacy

The victim can be reassured that the court process takes place in a private room at the court, which is not open to members of the public. The victim's solicitor will prepare a written statement for her to sign in support of her application for an injunction and/or occupation order. The victim will need to attend court when her application is heard. Special measures may be available to support and assist particularly vulnerable or intimidated witnesses (e.g. use of screens, giving evidence via a video link).

Standard of proof

The standard of proof is lower than in a criminal case. The court has to decide whether the allegations of violence are true on the balance of probabilities (in a criminal case, it must be beyond reasonable doubt).

Housing Acts 1985 and 1996

Under Ground 1 Schedule 2 of the Housing Act 1985, a possession order can be granted where an obligation of the tenancy has been broken or not performed. The Housing Act 1996 added Ground 2A of Schedule 2 to the Housing Act 1985. Under the Act, possession action can be taken against a remaining tenant where their partner has left the family home because of violence or threats of violence and does not intend to return. In such cases, sufficient evidence of violence having occurred is required, which can include evidence provided by any professional the victim is working with, such as a nurse or general practitioner. In addition, housing authorities can take injunctive action against a tenant if they are in breach of the terms of their tenancy agreement.

Other antisocial behaviour legislation also allows housing powers to act against perpetrators in respect of their tenancies. Practitioners should always seek advice from housing services when considering what options are available to the victim in securing protection for her and any children. It is good practice to invite housing officers to meetings arranged to draw up safety plans for victims.

Criminal action

The Crown Prosecution Service (2005) definition of domestic violence includes many forms of violent or controlling behaviour, illustrated in Table 6.1, with examples of the offences the perpetrator could be charged with.

Police officers are under a duty to take positive action when investigating domestic violence offences. There is an expectation that a perpetrator of domestic violence will be arrested in all criminal investigations where there are reasonable grounds to suspect that a crime has taken place. The power to arrest comes from Section 110 of the Serious Organised Crime and Police Act 2005, which amended the powers of arrest available to a

Table 6.1 Domestic violence examples from the Crown Prosecution Service (2005)

Examples of behaviour	Examples of possible offences
Pressuring the victim to 'drop the case'	Witness intimidation, obstructing the course of justice
Physical violence, e.g. punching, kicking, hair-pulling	Common assault, actual/grievous bodily harm, wounding, attempted murder
Violence resulting in miscarriage	Child destruction, procuring miscarriage
Threatening with an object used as a weapon, e.g. telephone	Threats to kill, common assault, affray, threatening behaviour
Throwing articles, e.g. crockery	Criminal damage, threatening behaviour
Stopping her seeing friends/family	False imprisonment, kidnapping, harassment
Racial abuse	Racially aggravated threatening behaviour, disorderly conduct, harassment
Dowry abuse	Blackmail, harassment, common assault
Constant criticism	Harassment, actual bodily harm
Forced marriage	Kidnap, blackmail, false imprisonment, common assault, indecent assault, rape
Abusive telephone calls	Malicious communications, improper use of public telecommunication systems
Excessive checking up on	Harassment, false imprisonment

constable under Section 24 of the Police and Criminal Evidence Act 1984. This has made all offences potentially arrestable in certain circumstances.

The exercise of arrest powers is subject to a 'necessity test', that is, an overriding requirement that an arrest is reasonably required and that no less intrusive way of advancing the investigation is reasonably available. When considering the need to arrest, the officer should take the following into account:

- the situation of the victim
- the nature of the offence
- the circumstances of the offender
- the needs of the investigation.

It is the role of the Crown Prosecution Service (CPS) to decide on whether a perpetrator should be charged with a criminal offence and what criminal offence(s) should be charged. If there is a disagreement between police and CPS, a dispute resolution process may be implemented to review charging decisions, although ultimately it is the CPS who has the final decision.

The typical offences (though this is not exhaustive) likely to be charged in domestic violence cases are listed in Table 6.2.

Of particular note are cases of homicide. British homicide statistics tell us that on average two women are killed every week by their current or former partner. Of these, one of the two will have already sought to escape their violent partner (Povey, 2005). The number of women killed by their partner

Table 6.2 Typical offences in domestic violence cases

Offences Against the Person Act 1861	
Section 18	Grievous bodily harm with intent
Section 20	Unintentional grievous bodily harm or wounding
Section 21	Attempted choking, strangulation and suffocation with intent to commit an indictable offence
Section 23	Administer poisonous/noxious substances with intent to endanger life
Section 47	Actual bodily harm
Protection from Harassment Act 1997	
Section 2/4	Harassment, fear of violence
Public Order Act 1986	
Section 3	Affray
Common law offences	
	Kidnap, unlawful imprisonment, breach of the peace

or ex-partner is approximately one in three, while the equivalent figure for men is approximately one in twelve. Until recently, women who killed their violent partners were faced with a stark choice: argue self-defence and risk conviction for murder (with a mandatory life sentence) or run a partial defence (either on the grounds of diminished responsibility or as a result of provocation), which would lead to a conviction for manslaughter rather than murder. Some viewed the law of provocation as biased against women in cases of domestic violence. The government's Solicitor General, Vera Baird, wrote in *The Guardian* in 2008 that the law is 'both too lenient on those who kill out of anger and too harsh on those who kill out of fear of violence'. The law was amended and the new provisions came into effect on 4 October 2010. The reforms apply to killings on or after that date. The common law defence of provocation was abolished and replaced by a new partial defence to be known as 'loss of control'. It no longer matters whether the killer's loss of self-control was sudden. It was postulated that this would make it 'the easier for the defence, particularly in respect of battered women, to run the slow-burn defence where a person has been subject to abuse over a long period of time when a final small act leads to the killing' (Edwards, 2010).

But defendants will still have to produce evidence that:

- the killing resulted from a loss of self-control;
- the loss of self-control had a 'qualifying trigger'; and
- a person in the same position 'with a normal degree of tolerance and self-restraint' might have reacted in a similar way.

A qualifying trigger can be: a fear of serious violence, or something said or done that was 'extremely grave' and gave the defendant 'a justifiable sense of being seriously wronged', or both (quotes from the Coroners and Justice Act 2009). In deciding whether the loss of self-control had a qualifying trigger, the courts must ignore such factors as sexual infidelity and a desire for revenge.

Since 2011, local community safety partnerships are required by law to initiate a multi-agency domestic homicide review following a killing in which domestic violence is suspected. This will involve all agencies which have had any contact with the victim, the victim's family or the perpetrator.

Statutory guidance has been issued under Section 9(3) of the Domestic Violence, Crime and Victims Act 2004. All public services, together with services which support victims of domestic violence, need to have a good understanding of the guidance and its requirements.

Giving evidence in court

It may be anxiety provoking, but it is important for professionals to give evidence in court, as such evidence can provide valuable and necessary information to the court. Professionals may find themselves in the witness box giving evidence on behalf of their organisation or in relation to a particular individual. Courts take many forms, and include tribunals (e.g. mental health tribunals, immigration tribunals), family proceedings courts, civil and criminal trials. Giving evidence can be a difficult and stressful experience; the English court system is adversarial and doubt may be cast on the practitioner's experience, notes and methods. This section outlines key elements in relation to giving evidence, the order of events and preparation for court appearance.

The adversarial system

The focus of this section is on criminal courts, and it is essential to remember that procedures in relation to civil courts and family courts are different and relate to different areas of law. The role and duties of witnesses in the different courts vary.

Generally, criminal proceedings involve a case which is brought by the State against a person accused of committing a crime, although in rare cases it is also possible to have a private prosecution. There are two forms of criminal trial in England and Wales: a summary trial and a trial on indictment. The former takes place in a magistrates' court and the latter in a Crown Court. Some offences can only be tried summarily, others only on indictment and some are triable either way. Summary offences tend to be the least serious offences, for example minor criminal damage or disorderly behaviour, whereas the indictable-only offences are the most serious, for example murder or rape. There are two types of principal criminal courts in England and Wales, the magistrates' court and the Crown Court. About 97% of cases are disposed of in the magistrates' court, whereas the Crown Court deals with more serious and complex cases.

The criminal proceedings are conducted in accordance with the Criminal Procedure Rules 2010. These rules came into effect on 5 April 2010 and apply to all cases in the magistrates' court, the Crown Court and the criminal division of the Court of Appeal.

The central role of the court is to act as an unbiased arbiter, deciding which of two (or more) conflicting versions of events or arguments it favours. Witnesses will give evidence, having been called by one party's lawyer and will then be cross-examined by the lawyers of the opposing party. Although giving evidence can be intimidating, clinicians should always remember that they are there to assist the court and to explain their findings or opinion. It may be the barrister who asks the questions but the clinician's answers should be directed not to them but to the judge and jury.

Types of witness

There are three types of witness:
1   Witness to fact: a person with knowledge about what happened in a particular case, who testifies about what happened or what the facts are; gives their full name only.

2   Professional witness: presents primary rather than expert evidence from a professional perspective; gives their full name and professional address.

3   Expert witness: a person who is a specialist in a subject, who may present his/her expert opinion without having been a witness to any occurrence relating to the case; gives their full name and address as it appears on their report and gives their qualifications and relevant experience.

Procedure in the witness box

You will be asked to swear, to take the oath, or affirm. It is important to do this solemnly and clearly. This is a useful time to 'test' your voice, and think about the pace and volume of your speech. If you swear, you will be asked to take the holy book in your uplifted right hand and read the oath from a card. Those affirming must just read the words from the card. Both the oath and the affirmation carry the same weight and you commit perjury if you lie after this point.

Questioning

Examination-in-Chief (also known as direct examination)

The lawyer who called you as a witness will ask you questions first. It is likely that they will start by asking you your name, position and experience; make sure that you are clear in your answers. They will then move on to your evidence. Listen to each question and take your time to answer. Be familiar with your evidence and make sure that you have re-read your report or case notes before giving evidence. Make your answers easy to understand.

Cross-examination

Next, the lawyers for the other 'side' will have the opportunity to question you. These lawyers are likely to be trying to undermine what you have already said and it is important to think on your feet and be aware of their techniques. Take your time to answer. If you need clarification, request this through the judge. Do not stray outside your remit. Do not defend the indefensible. Always remember that your role as a witness is to help the court come to a decision by answering questions. You need to give complete answers and not mislead. Think clearly about the points that you want to make and be sure to make them. Do not be railroaded by lawyers into giving half an answer to a question or answering something that you do not know the answer to. You can say you do not know and refuse to speculate.

Re-examination

The lawyer who first asked you questions will sometimes ask further questions to clarify matters that have arisen out of the cross-examination.

If there is a break in the middle of your evidence, for example for lunch or at the end of the day, remember that you are not free to discuss the case with anyone including your lawyers until you have completed your evidence and been released by the judge.

What to call judges and lawyers

This often worries people. The rules are complex and certain courts and roles are excluded from the normal rules. The simplest solution to this is to ask the barrister or the clerk of the court before you enter court who is hearing the case and how you should refer to them.

In general terms, in the magistrates', youth and family proceedings courts and in tribunals the person in charge should be referred to as 'Sir' or 'Madam', and those sitting with them as 'your colleagues'. In the county court all but district judges are referred to as 'Your Honour', with district judges referred to as 'Sir' or 'Madam'. In the Crown Court circuit judges and recorders are generally referred to as 'Your Honour' and High Court judges or anyone sitting at the Central Criminal Court as 'My Lord' or 'My Lady'. In the High Court all judges are referred to as 'My Lord' or 'My Lady'.

Practical suggestions

It is vital to be prepared before giving evidence in court. Good preparation will reduce your stress levels significantly. It may help to consider the points listed here:

(a)   In relation to your evidence:
- Re-read your notes and statement or report.
  - If you find errors in your statement or report, note them and bring them to the attention of your instructing lawyer. It is better to be prepared to address these rather than waiting to be confronted about them during cross-examination.
- Prepare the documents that you will take with you, including your contemporaneous notes. Make sure they are organised and you can find all documents easily. Use indexing to assist you.
- Identify all the essential issues in your evidence, and think through what you may be asked. In particular, think of the questions that you do not want to be asked and make sure you are clear how to answer those.
- Be clear about the key points that you wish to communicate to the court. It is well worth thinking this through in advance, and it may be helpful to highlight these on your report or to write a summary that you can review before giving evidence.
- Make sure you have prepared clear explanations for any terminology that may not be easily understood.

(b)   In relation to practical arrangements:
- Visit a court before giving evidence for the first time and watch another hearing.

- Check the timing of the court hearing and when you are expected to be there.
- Get contact details for those who will be meeting at court.
- Find out where the court is.
- Wear a dark suit.
- Leave plenty of time and, if necessary, travel the day before if you are likely to be called first thing.
- Make sure you have travel arrangements (including car parking) and accommodation arrangements in hand.
- Arrange a meeting point with those who instructed you.
- Clarify the status of the judge and the right form of address.
- Take something to do while waiting.
- Be prepared to wait, potentially for a long time (on rare occasions, this can take up days).

(c) In the witness box:

- Direct your answers to the decision maker, not the person questioning you.
- As soon as you enter the witness box, stand with your feet pointing towards the judge. Do not then move your feet, but instead turn to look at those questioning you, or the jury, when appropriate.
- Face the questioning lawyer by turning. When the question is finished, turn back to face the judge before giving your answer.
- Do not engage in an argument with the lawyer; address any queries to the judge.
- Watch the judge, who may be making notes by hand. You want the judge to be able to keep up with your evidence. If you wait for them to finish writing they will then be able to listen to the next part of your answer. This will also give you time to think about what you are going to say next.
- If there is a jury, direct your answers to both the judge and the jury.[1]
- Only sit down if invited to do so. Consider remaining standing even if you are invited to sit down.
- Try to control the pace; this is easier if you do not turn and look at the lawyer until you are ready for the next question.
- Remember that you have been called to assist the court. Take your time, do not get flustered and stick to your area of expertise.

---

1   Note you do not address the jury directly. The point is not to feel that you have to direct your answers at the barrister who asked the question. It is about where you look when answering, and not a verbal form of address. The feet positioning means that you are naturally pointing towards the judge, and with only a slight turn will be looking at the jury.

References

Association of Directors of Social Services (2005) *Safeguarding Adults: A National Framework of Standards for Good Practice and Outcomes in Adult Protection Work.* ADSS.

Baird, V. (2008) Bringing homicide law up to date. *Guardian,* 5 August.

British Medical Association (2011) *Safeguarding Vulnerable Adults – A Toolkit for General Practitioners.* BMA.

Brownridge, D. (2006) Partner violence against women with disabilities: prevalence, risk and explanations. *Violence Against Women,* **12,** 805–822.

Crown Prosecution Service (2005) *Policy for Prosecuting Cases of Domestic Violence.* CPS Policy Directorate.

Department of Health (2000) *No Secrets: Guidance on Developing and Implementing Multi-Agency Policies and Procedures to Protect Vulnerable Adults from Abuse.* Department of Health.

Department of Health (2002) *Women's Mental Health: Into the Mainstream. Strategic Development of Mental Health Care for Women.* Department of Health.

Department of Health (2008) *Refocusing the Care Programme Approach: Policy and Positive Practice Guidance.* Department of Health.

Edleson, J. L. (1999) The overlap between child maltreatment and woman battering. *Violence Against Women,* **5,** 134–154.

Edwards, A. (2010) Changes to the law of homicide. *Law Society Gazette,* 2 September.

Hester, M., Pearson, C. & Harwin, N. (2000) *Making an Impact: A Reader.* Jessica Kingsley Publishers.

HM Government (2004) *Every Child Matters: Change for Children.* DfES Publications.

HM Government (2010) *Working Together to Safeguard Children: A Guide to Inter-Agency Working to Safeguard and Promote the Welfare of Children.* DCSF Publications.

Humphreys, C. & Thiara, R. (2002) *Routes to Safety: Protection Issues Facing Abused Women and Children and the Role of Outreach Services.* Women's Aid Federation of England.

Lord Chancellor's Department (1997) *Who Decides: Making Decisions on Behalf of Mentally Incapacitated Adults; A Consultation Paper Issued by the Lord Chancellor's Department; Presented to Parliament by the Lord High Chancellor by Command of Her Majesty December 1997.* TSO (The Stationery Office).

O'Keefe, M., Hills, A., Doyle, M., *et al* (2007) *UK Study of Abuse and Neglect of Older People: Prevalence Survey Report.* Department of Health.

Povey, D. (2005) *Crime in England and Wales 2003/2004: Supplementary Volume 1: Homicide and Gun Crime.* Home Office Statistical Bulletin No. 02/05.

Royal College of Psychiatrists (2013) Domestic violence: its effects on children. In *Mental Health and Growing Up: Factsheets for Parents, Teachers and Young People* (4th edn). RCPsych Publications.

Trevillion, K., Howard, L.M., Morgan, C., *et al* (2012) The response of mental health services to domestic violence: a qualitative study of service users' and professionals' experiences. *Journal of the American Psychiatric Nurses Association,* epub ahead of print, doi: 10.1177/1078390312459747.

L. v. Sweden (1988) Application no. 10801/84,61 Eur. Comm'n H.R. Dec. & Rep. 62, 73.

Relevant UK and European legislation and guidelines

Adoption and Children Act 2002

Children Act 1989

Children Act 2004

Coroners and Justice Act 2009

Department for Constitutional Affairs (2007) *Mental Capacity Act 2005 Code of Practice.* TSO (The Stationery Office)

Domestic Violence, Crime and Victims Act 2004

European Convention on Human Rights 1950
Housing Act 1985
Housing Act 1996
Human Rights Act 1998
Mental Capacity Act 2005
Mental Health Act 1983
Police and Criminal Evidence Act 1984
Serious Organised Crime and Police Act 2005

Additional reading

Here are links to some good practice materials that underpin the current UK government's approach to safeguarding.

Department of Health, 2010: *A Vision for Adult Social Care: Capable Communities and Active Citizens* (http://webarchive.nationalarchives.gov.uk/+/www.dh.gov.uk/en/Publicationsandstatistics/Publications/PublicationsPolicyAndGuidance/DH_121508).

Department of Health, 2010: *Practical Approaches to Safeguarding and Personalisation* (http://www.dh.gov.uk/en/Publicationsandstatistics/Lettersandcirculars/LocalAuthorityCirculars/DH_131569).

Department of Health, 2011: *Transparency in Outcomes: A Framework for Quality in Adult Social Care – Response to Consultation* (http://www.dh.gov.uk/en/Consultations/Responsestoconsultations/DH_125464).

Department of Health, 2011: *Safeguarding Adults: The Role of Health Services*, guidance for managers, commissioners and nurses (http://www.dh.gov.uk/en/Publicationsandstatistics/Publications/PublicationsPolicyAndGuidance/DH_124882).

Department of Health, 2011: *Safeguarding Adults: The Role of Health Services*, a guide to achieving good outcomes in safeguarding adults in health services, with a voluntary self-assessment framework (http://www.dh.gov.uk/en/Publicationsandstatistics/Publications/PublicationsPolicyAndGuidance/DH_124882).

Howard, L. M., Trevillion, K. & Agnew–Davies, R. (2010) Domestic violence and mental health. *International Review of Psychiatry*, **22**, 525–534.

Local Government Association, 2011: *Standards for Adult Safeguarding: Standards and Probes for Adult Safeguarding Peer Reviews* (www.local.gov.uk).

Social Care Institute for Excellence and Pan London Adult Safeguarding Editorial Board, 2011: *Protecting Adults at Risk: London Multi-Agency Policy and Procedures to Safeguard Adults from Abuse* (http://www.scie.org.uk/publications/reports/report39.pdf).

Appendix 1: CAADA Risk Identification Checklist (RIC) and Quick Start Guidance for Domestic Abuse, Stalking and 'Honour'-Based Violence[†]

†Adapted from the CAADA Domestic Abuse, Stalking and 'Honour'-Based Violence Risk Identification Checklist. The full list is available at www.caada.org.uk/marac/RIC_with_guidance.pdf and should only be used in conjunction with the introductory notes.

Abbreviations used in the checklist:
ACPO, Association of Chief Police Officers; DV, domestic violence; HBV, 'honour'-based violence; IDVAs, independent domestic violence advocates; MARAC, Multi-Agency Risk Assessment Conference.

The DASH 2009 risk assessment model is the Domestic Abuse, Stalking and Harassment and 'Honour'-Based Violence (DASH, 2009) Risk Identification and Assessment and Management Model, available from www.dashriskchecklist.co.uk

CAADA-DASH Risk Identification Checklist for use by IDVAs and other non-police agencies[3] for MARAC case identification when domestic abuse, 'honour'-based violence and/or stalking are disclosed

Please explain that the purpose of asking these questions is for the safety and protection of the individual concerned. Tick the box if the factor is present ☑. Please use the comment box at the end of the form to expand on any answer. It is assumed that your main source of information is the victim. If this is *not the case* please indicate in the right hand column	Yes (tick)	No	Don't know	State source of info if not the victim e.g. police officer
1. Has the current incident resulted in injury? (Please state what and whether this is the first injury.)	☐	☐	☐	
2. Are you very frightened? Comment:	☐	☐	☐	
3. What are you afraid of? Is it further injury or violence? (Please give an indication of what you think (name of abuser(s) ....) might do and to whom, including children.) Comment:	☐	☐	☐	
4. Do you feel isolated from family/friends i.e. does (...........) try to stop you from seeing friends/family/ doctor or others? Comment:	☐	☐	☐	
5. Are you feeling depressed or having suicidal thoughts?	☐	☐	☐	
6. Have you separated or tried to separate from (...........) within the past year?	☐	☐	☐	
7. Is there conflict over child contact?	☐	☐	☐	
8. Does (...........) constantly text, call, contact, follow, stalk or harass you? (Please expand to identify what and whether you believe that this is done deliberately to intimidate you? Consider the context and behaviour of what is being done.)	☐	☐	☐	
9. Are you pregnant or have you recently had a baby (within the past 18 months)?	☐	☐	☐	
10. Is the abuse happening more often?	☐	☐	☐	
11. Is the abuse getting worse?	☐	☐	☐	
12. Does (...........) try to control everything you do and/or are they excessively jealous? (In terms of relationships, who you see, being 'policed at home', telling you what to wear for example. Consider 'honour'-based violence and specify behaviour.)	☐	☐	☐	
13. Has (...........) ever used weapons or objects to hurt you?	☐	☐	☐	

3   This checklist is consistent with the ACPO endorsed risk assessment model DASH 2009 for the police service.

Tick the box if the factor is present ☑. Please use the comment box at the end of the form to expand on any answer.	Yes	No	Don't know	Source of info if not the victim
14. Has (............) ever threatened to kill you or someone else and you believed them? (If yes, tick who.) You☐ Children☐ Other (please specify)☐	☐	☐	☐	
15. Has (............) ever attempted to strangle/choke/suffocate/drown you?	☐	☐	☐	
16. Does (............) do or say things of a sexual nature that make you feel bad or that physically hurt you or someone else? (If someone else, specify who.)	☐	☐	☐	
17. Is there any other person who has threatened you or who you are afraid of? (If yes, please specify whom and why. Consider extended family if HBV.)	☐	☐	☐	
18. Do you know if (............) has hurt anyone else? (Please specify whom including the children, siblings or elderly relatives. Consider HBV.) Children☐ Another family member☐ Someone from a previous relationship☐ Other (please specify)☐	☐	☐	☐	
19. Has (............) ever mistreated an animal or the family pet?	☐	☐	☐	
20. Are there any financial issues? For example, are you dependent on (............) for money/have they recently lost their job/other financial issues?	☐	☐	☐	
21. Has (............) had problems in the past year with drugs (prescription or other), alcohol or mental health leading to problems in leading a normal life? (If yes, please specify which and give relevant details if known.) Drugs☐ Alcohol☐ Mental health☐	☐	☐	☐	
22. Has (............) ever threatened or attempted suicide?	☐	☐	☐	
23. Has (............) ever broken bail/an injunction and/or formal agreement for when they can see you and/or the children? (You may wish to consider this in relation to an ex-partner of the perpetrator if relevant.) Bail conditions☐ Non Molestation/Occupation Order☐ Child Contact arrangements☐ Forced Marriage Protection Order☐ Other☐	☐	☐	☐	
24. Do you know if (............) has ever been in trouble with the police or has a criminal history? (If yes, please specify.) DV☐ Sexual violence☐ Other violence☐ Other☐	☐	☐	☐	
Total 'yes' responses				

For consideration by professional: Is there any other relevant information (from victim or professional) which may increase risk levels? Consider victim's situation in relation to disability, substance misuse, mental health issues, cultural/language barriers, 'honour'-based systems, geographic isolation and minimisation. Are they willing to engage with your service? Describe:

Consider abuser's occupation/interests — could this give them unique access to weapons? Describe:

What are the victim's greatest priorities to address their safety?

Do you believe that there are reasonable grounds for referring this case to MARAC? Yes / No
If yes, have you made a referral? Yes / No

Signed: .... Date: ....

Do you believe that there are risks facing the children in the family? Yes / No
If yes, please confirm if you have made a referral to safeguard the children: Yes / No

Date referral made: ....

Signed: .... Date: ....

Name: ....

Practitioner's notes:

Appendix 2: Domestic violence resources and directory of services

Resources

Against Violence and Abuse (www.avaproject.org.uk):
- *The Coordinated Community Response to Domestic Violence Toolkit*: www.ccrm.org.uk
- *Sane Responses: Good Practice Guidelines for Domestic Violence and Mental Health Services* (2008), available on the AVA website

Barron, J. (2005) *Health and Domestic Volence – Good Practice Guidelines. Principles of Good Practice for Working with Women Experiencing Domestic Violence (Guidance for Mental Health Professionals)* available at www.womensaid.org.uk

British Medical Association (http://bma.org.uk):
- *Victims of Forced Marriage: Guidance for Health Professionals* (2008) available on the BMA website
- *Domestic Abuse: A Report from the BMA Board of Science* (eds S. How & N. Jayesinghe, 2007), can be requested from the British Library

Co-ordinated Action Against Domestic Abuse (CAADA):
- *Resources for Practitioners who Refer to Multi-Agency Risk Assessment Conferences (MARACs)*: www.caada.org.uk/marac/Resources_for_people_who_refer_to_MARAC.html

Department of Health (www.dh.gov.uk):
- *No Secrets: Guidance on Developing and Implementing Multi-Agency Policies and Procedures to Protect Vulnerable Adults from Abuse* (2000)
- *Responding to Domestic Abuse: A Handbook for Health Professionals* (2005)
- *Improving Safety, Reducing Harm: Children, Young People and Domestic Violence* (2009)
- *Responding to Violence against Women and Children – The Role of the NHS* (2010)

Ethnic Alcohol Counselling in Hounslow (EACH):
- *Asian Women, Domestic Violence and Mental Health: A Toolkit for Health Professionals* (2009): http://ndvf.org.uk/files/document/817/original.pdf

Home Office (www.homeoffice.gov.uk):

- *Tackling Domestic Violence: The Role of Health Professionals* (2nd edn) (2004). This report can be found in the research and statistics section of the Home Office website (www.homeoffice.gov.uk/science-research/research-statistics)

National Institute for Health and Clinical Excellence (NICE):

- *Preventing and Reducing Domestic Violence.* This guidance is still in development, but useful information can be accessed at http://guidance.nice.org.uk/PHG/44

PreVAil: Preventing Violence Across the Lifespan Research Network (www.prevailresearch.ca)

Royal College of Psychiatrists (www.rcpsych.ac.uk):

- *Domestic Violence – Its Effects on Children: The Impact on Children and Adolescents: Information for Parents, Carers and Anyone who Works with Young People* (2012). This factsheet is available on the Expert advice: Youth info section of the College's website.

Social Care Institute for Excellence (SCIE):

- Sexual, reproductive and mental health e-learning programme for mental health practitioners. Module 3: Supporting clients who experience abuse, available at www.scie.org.uk/assets/elearning/sexualhealth/Web/Object3/main.html

UNICEF (www.unicef.org):

- *Behind Closed Doors: The Impact of Domestic Violence on Children* (2006). A report that was part of a UK campaign against violence, Stop Violence in the Home, available at www.unicef.org/protection/files/BehindClosedDoors.pdf

World Health Organization (www.who.int):

- Intimate partner and sexual violence prevention course. A course developed by the WHO for individuals engaged in child maltreatment prevention and supporting victims of intimate partner and sexual violence in a wide range of capacities. Course materials can be downloaded from www.who.int/violence_injury_prevention/capacitybuilding/courses/intimate_partner_violence/en/index.html
- *Preventing Intimate Partner Violence and Sexual Violence against Women: Taking Action and Generating Evidence* (2010). A report from the WHO and London School of Hygiene and Tropical Medicine, available at www.who.int/violence_injury_prevention/publications/violence/9789241564007_eng.pdf
- *Guidelines for Medico-Legal Care for Victims of Sexual Violence* (2003) http://whqlibdoc.who.int/publications/2004/924154628X.pdf

Support services for female victims of domestic violence

In an emergency always phone 999.

Refuge

Refuge provides emergency accommodation for women and children, outreach projects, individual and group counselling, and children's services for those fleeing domestic violence.

Free 24-hour National Domestic Violence Helpline, run by Refuge in partnership with Women's Aid: 0808 2000 247

www.refuge.org.uk

National Centre for Domestic Violence (NCDV)

Provides free, fast injunctions for anyone experiencing domestic violence.

Telephone: 0844 8044 999

www.ncdv.org.uk

Women's Aid Federation of England

Women's Aid coordinates an England-wide network of over 500 local services and offers support, advice and information on all aspects of domestic violence.

Free 24-hour National Domestic Violence Helpline, run by Women's Aid in partnership with Refuge: 0808 2000 247

www.womensaid.org.uk

Rights of Women

Free confidential legal advice for women on domestic violence, harassment and divorce. Also offers advice on sexual offences, child contact and residence, trafficking and the criminal justice system.

General and family law advice line: 020 7251 6577 (Monday 11am–1pm, Tuesday & Wednesday 2pm–4pm and 7pm–9pm, Thursday 7pm–9pm, Friday 12pm–2pm)

Criminal law and sexual violence legal advice line: 020 7251 8887 (Tuesday 11am–1pm, Thursday 2pm–4pm)

Immigration and asylum legal advice line: 020 7490 7689 (Monday 2pm–4pm, Wednesday 11am–1pm)

www.rightsofwomen.org.uk

Advocacy after Fatal Domestic Abuse (AAFDA)

Support, information and advocacy for families who have suffered fatal (or near-fatal) domestic violence.

If you need immediate assistance call: 07768 386922 (Monday–Friday 9am–5pm)

Email: info@aafda.org.uk

www.aafda.org.uk

Victim Support Helpline

Emotional support and information for victims of crime.
Helpline: 0845 30 30 900 (Monday–Friday 9am–9pm, weekends 9am–7pm)
www.victimsupport.org.uk

Rape and Sexual Abuse Support Centre (RASASC)

National helpline providing emotional support and practical information
to survivors (aged 14+ years) of rape or childhood sexual abuse. The
helpline also offers information to family, friends, partners of survivors
and professionals.
Freephone helpline: 0808 802 9999 (line open every day between 12pm–
2.30pm and 7pm–9.30pm)
Counselling/advocacy: 0208 683 3311
http://rasasc.bizview.co.uk

Action on Elder Abuse

National helpline for anyone concerned about the abuse of older people.
Free helpline UK: 0808 808 8141
Free helpline Ireland: 1800 940 010
www.elderabuse.org.uk

Voice UK

Supports people with intellectual disabilities who are victims of crime or
abuse, their families, carers and professional workers.
Free helpline: 0808 802 8686
www.voiceuk.org.uk

Support services for male victims of domestic violence

In an emergency always phone 999.

Mankind

Support for male victims of domestic violence and abuse.
Confidential helpline: 01823 334 244 (Monday–Friday 10am–4pm and
7pm–9pm)
www.mankind.org.uk

Survivors UK

Information, support and counselling for male survivors of sexual abuse
and rape.
Telephone: 0845 122 1201 (Monday & Tuesday 7pm–9.30pm, Thursday
12pm–2.30pm)
www.survivorsuk.org

Men's Advice Line

A service run by Respect. Provides support for male victims and information and counselling for men experiencing domestic violence; telephone advice line; face-to-face outreach work; liaison with other services.
Free helpline: 0808 801 0327 (Monday–Friday 10am–1pm and 2pm–5pm)
www.mensadviceline.org.uk

Respect Phoneline

A service for perpetrators of domestic violence and front-line workers.
Free helpline: 0808 802 4040 (Monday–Friday 10am–1pm and 2–5pm)
www.respectphoneline.org.uk

Samaritans

A service that provides confidential emotional support (via telephone or email) for people who are experiencing feelings of distress, despair or having suicidal thoughts.
24-hour service (automatic transfer to local branch)
UK: 08457 90 90 90
Ireland: 1850 60 90 90
www.samaritans.org.uk

And also:

National Centre for Domestic Violence (NCDV)
Advocacy after Fatal Domestic Abuse (AAFDA)
Victim Support Helpline
Action on Elder Abuse
Voice UK
For contact details, see pp. 104–105.

Helplines for mothers and fathers

In an emergency always phone 999.

National Society for the Prevention of Cruelty to Children (NSPCC)

Helpline for anyone concerned a child may be at risk.
24-hour free helpline: 0808 800 5000
www.nspcc.org.uk

Parentline

Provides helpline support, advice and information to anyone looking after a child and offers extended support for complex and difficult issues.
Confidential helpline: 0808 800 2222 (open every day from 7am until midnight)
Text-phone: 0800 783 6783
www.familylives.org.uk

Barnardo's

Barnardo's provides advice and information to young people and their families, counselling for children who have been abused, fostering and adoption services, vocational training and disability inclusion groups.
Head office telephone: 020 8550 8822
www.barnardos.org.uk

Reunite International Child Abduction Centre

Advice and support to parents or families who fear or experience child abduction.
Advice line: 0116 2556 234
Telephone: 0116 2556 235
www.reunite.org

Support services for lesbian, gay, bisexual and transgender victims of domestic violence

In an emergency always phone 999.

Broken Rainbow

Support for lesbian, gay, bisexual and transgender people experiencing domestic violence.
Helpline: 0300 999 5428 (Monday & Thursday 10am–8pm, Tuesday & Wednesday 10am–5pm; Tuesday 1pm–5pm service specifically for transgender people)
www.broken-rainbow.org.uk

Alternative Family Law

Source of information on family law in families with lesbian, gay, bisexual and transgender people.
www.alternativefamilylaw.co.uk

And also:

Victim Support Helpline
Action on Elder Abuse
Voice UK
Samaritans
Parentline
For contact details, see pp. 105–106.

Support services for ethnic and religious minority victims of domestic violence

In an emergency always phone 999.

Karma Nirvana

Support for victims and survivors of forced marriages and 'honour'-based violence.
Honour network helpline: 0800 5999 247
www.karmanirvana.org.uk

Ashiana Project

Provides advice, support and safe temporary housing for young South Asian, Turkish and Iranian women escaping abuse (aged 16–30 without children).
Telephone: 020 8539 0427, 020 8539 9656 (Monday–Friday 9.30am–5pm)
www.ashiana.org.uk

Akina Mama Wa Afrika

Provides advice, information, counselling, lectures and workshops for young African women (25–45 years) covering domestic violence, HIV/AIDS and mental health.
www.akinamamawaafrika.org

Jewish Women's Aid Helpline

Advice and support for Jewish women and children experiencing domestic violence.
Freephone helpline: 0808 801 0500 (Monday–Thursday 9.30am–9.30pm)
www.jwa.org.uk

The Foreign and Commonwealth Office's Forced Marriage Unit

Caseworkers dedicated to preventing British nationals being forced into marriage overseas.
Confidential helpline: 020 7008 0151
www.fco.gov.uk/en/travel-and-living-abroad/when-things-go-wrong/forced-marriage/

And also:

Samaritans
For contact details, see p. 106.

Support services for children and young people living with domestic violence

In an emergency always phone 999.

ChildLine

Confidential counselling service for children with any sort of problems, provided by the NSPCC.
Free 24-hour helpline: 0800 1111
Children can also chat to a counsellor, send an email or post a message on one of the website's message boards.
www.childline.org.uk

The Hide Out

Run by Women's Aid, this website provides a space to help children and young people understand about domestic violence and to take positive action if they are affected by it.
www.thehideout.org.uk

National Youth Advocacy Service (NYAS)

A national charity providing social and legal advice, support and representation for children, young people and vulnerable adults.
Free helpline: 0300 330 3131 (weekdays 9am–8pm, Saturday 10am–4pm)
Email: help@nyas.net
www.nyas.net

HOPELineUK

A helpline service that provides advice and information for children and young people up to the age of 35 in emotional distress, and those worried about them.
Confidential helpline (free for landline calls): 0800 068 41 41 (Monday–Friday 10am–5pm and 7pm–10pm, weekends 2pm–5pm)
Email: pat@papyrus-uk.org
SMS: 07786 209697
www.papyrus-uk.org/more/hopelineuk

And also:

National Society for the Prevention of Cruelty to Children (NSPCC)
Barnardo's
For contact details, see pp. 106–107.

Index

Compiled by Linda English